Alkaline Soups

Quick & Easy, Delicious, Creamy & Nutritious Alkaline (and Almost Alkaline) Recipes to Help You Look & Feel Amazing

By Marta "Wellness" Tuchowska

IMPORTANT

This book is not intended to provide medical advice or to take the place of medical advice and treatment from your personal physician. Readers are advised to consult their own doctors or other qualified health professionals regarding the treatment of medical conditions. The author shall not be held liable or responsible for any misunderstanding or misuse of the information contained in this book. The information is not intended to diagnose, treat, or cure any disease.

It is important to remember that the author of this book is not a doctor/ medical professional. Only opinions based upon her own personal experiences or research are cited. THE AUTHOR DOES NOT OFFER MEDICAL ADVICE or prescribe any treatments. For any health or medical issues – you should be talking to your doctor first.

Contents

Introduction to the World of Delicious, Creamy and Super Nutritious Alkaline Soups

Thank you so much for taking an interest in this book. I am very excited for you because I know it has the potential to revolutionize your health and improve your wellbeing.

Alkaline soups are made of nutrient-dense, energy-packed and balance-stimulating superfoods to help you restore your energy levels and give your body what it needs to thrive.

And they are just perfect for people who are looking for easy recipes that are healthy and can be made even on a busy schedule.

Even if right now, you are totally new to the world of healthy, clean food eating, the alkaline diet, and lifestyle, don't worry. I will take you by the hand and show you exactly what steps you need to take so that you can focus on creating sustainable results without feeling overwhelmed.

If you are already an alkaline veteran, I am confident my book will provide you with a plethora of ideas to help you reach new exciting goals on your wellness quest.

This guide is written as a practical and easy to follow manual for a busy person who is health-conscious, values their wellbeing but doesn't have the time for overcomplicating their wellness rituals or deciphering complicated nutrition information.

The good news is: Simplicity means wellness.

I believe that alkaline soups genuinely hold power to solve many challenges and problems that people on the Alkaline Diet lifestyle or any healthy lifestyle might have, such as:

- *"I want to eat healthier, but I don't have the time to cook healthy food all the time."*

- *"I tried blending some veggies into raw soups. I really did my best, but the ones I tried didn't taste nice. Can I actually make something healthy and alkaline-rich that also tastes good?"*

- *"I wanted to try a healthy lifestyle, but I was advised to buy all those expensive powders and supplements. Is there a simpler way to make healthy, alkaline recipes?"*

-*"I really wanted to give this alkaline thing a try, but I didn't know who to listen to, and after doing some online research, my head was spinning. I am still not too sure which foods are actually alkaline or what the point of this diet is."*

- *"I like living a healthy lifestyle, but when I am stressed, I tend to get off track, is there a way to control my motivation?"*

The last one is one of my favorites. I am very passionate about the mindset. I love teaching people how to set their minds for long-term wellness success so that they no longer feel like living a healthy lifestyle has to be a struggle.
In alignment with that, all of my books and articles- even simple recipe guides like this one- are carefully infused with

my tested, love-based, unshakable mindset and motivation techniques.

I want you to stay confident in your healthy actions and LOVE your journey!

No more feeling like you "can't stick to it," or "maybe you will start next week."

Once you discover the mind-body energizing benefits of alkaline foods (in this case – alkaline soups), you will naturally crave more and more of all the good stuff. And since this is not a strict diet book, you can relax, enjoy the journey and focus on one small step at a time.

The goal is to create a healthy, alkaline-inspired lifestyle you love. The lifestyle that fits you, your nutritional preferences, your schedule, and your personal needs.

The soup recipes I share in this book are rich in clean protein, healthy fiber, and good fats that will help you stay full for hours.

A fresh alkaline soup for lunch will help you stay energized in the afternoon and avoid sugar / crappy carb temptations.

It's not even about "staying full" as the primary goal. The main goal is to stay nourished, energized, and balanced.

When that state of optimal wellness is achieved, your body no longer lacks nutrients. Because of that, it can pay you back with vibrant health and energy. You feel more focused and happier. When you give yourself permission to experience such a state, you actually crave more and more health, and you genuinely enjoy healthy eating and conscious living.

Even a small serving of a nutrient-packed, delicious alkaline soup with your main meal can help you feel more energized...

The main message that I always share with my beloved Readers is – first focus on ADDING. The rest becomes so much easier!

This book will show you the art of adding more clean and alkaline foods to your diet using the art of alkaline soups.

Yes, alkaline soups are the primary guest at our Alkaline Wellness party! They finally got an entire book dedicated to them, and they are so happy about it! (other books in this series include Alkaline Teas, Alkaline Salads, Alkaline Protein Smoothies, Alkaline Juicing...oh, and Alkaline Smoothie Bowls!).

People always ask me how I stay energized to write so many books.

And I always tell them -*Well, I eat my own dog food, lol!*

I mean – alkaline food, drinks, and lifestyle. Not that I am super perfect with it. But, most of my diet (about 80%) is alkaline-friendly, and this is what keeps me going as far as my physical and mental energy is concerned.

I have also taught my methodology of alkaline living to many high performers, high achievers, entrepreneurs, and bestselling authors who, after experiencing all the amazing benefits of alkaline-rich recipes, simply can't live without alkaline foods.

They feel so much more focused, efficient, and productive. The reason why I mention this is that it's not only about weight loss. Well, yes, you can experience natural weight loss as a side effect of living more alkaline. It's totally possible. But, aside from assisting you in transforming your body, alkaline foods, drinks, and lifestyle can also help you enjoy more energy for life.

And you can use this energy to transform all areas of your life.

Think of it as a bigger picture. Your why. And your deep MOTIVATION!

I wish I could just write a “nutrition-nutrition” cookie-cutter book or just a "recipe-recipe" book. Still, I swear to God, I always get off-topic and start writing about mindset, motivation, and the bigger picture.

Some people may not be ready for it. Still, I genuinely believe that by connecting to your deeper WHY and aligning your health and wellness goals, with all areas of your life, you can truly transform your self-image and your confidence.

You can become a totally new person. And it will feel so normal and natural to you! You are just someone who ENJOYS healthy eating and living. You just do it. You LOVE nourishing your body, mind, and soul with super delicious alkaline foods. You don't even need motivation. It's so normal, it's who you are, and you just love the process!

So, please declare your commitment. I know you are busy. And so, the best thing you can do is to commit to small, daily micro-goals. For example, I have very dedicated Alkaline Readers, who got one of my previous books (for instance *Alkaline Protein Smoothies*), and their commitment is to make one alkaline smoothie a day (the focus is on adding, I am not saying they live on alkaline smoothies alone, lol!).

So, are you committed to adding?

What is your plan? Are you excited? As you go through this book, share your commitment and experience with other readers by posting a review. Many people may get inspired by it!

It's really that simple. The simplest thing you could ever do. When you focus on adding (you don't have to be super perfect), healthy living will become so much easier.

By adding more alkaline foods to your diet, you will give your body the nourishment it needs to help you thrive. You see, all those unwanted food cravings are, most likely, the result of not giving your body what it needs. You may feed it some calories. But are these calories coming from healthy, clean, and nutritious, unprocessed food? Or processed food that makes you sick, tired, and doesn't align with your health goals?

More good news for you, my friend! By adding more "good stuff" into your diet, letting go of what no longer serves you (or reducing it), will become so much easier and more "automatic."

It all starts with this simple commitment- adding. Focus on adding.

So, before we really get this Alkaline Soup party going, please take a piece of paper and write down- yes, write it down...

I am committed to, and I am focused on adding more alkaline foods into my diet...!

Use it to stay motivated. Use it to keep going. Use it to make healthier choices as much as you can!

Healthy choices attract more health. A profound transformation is created by those small actions, taken daily. It's not about being 100% perfect every day.

Also, please note, this book, alkaline diet, and alkaline soups are not only for vegans, vegetarians, alkaline-freaks, or "plant-based-tarians." I welcome you all. Whatever diet you follow, I am confident you can add alkaline soups as a tool to your health and wellness toolbox.

Also, this book is not a strict diet book, nor a cleanse book. Be free to pick and choose the tips and recipes you feel can help you at the current stage of your journey. Focus on adding an abundance of nutrient-packed alkaline foods and drinks to your diet.

This mindset is so liberating, isn't it? Most diet books start off with, "Get rid of this, don't eat that." And yes, needless to say, to live a healthy lifestyle we need to let go of unhealthy habits.

However, this is so much easier to achieve when we allow ourselves to focus on abundance first.

In this book, you'll find no bashing, no nutritional dogmas, no dietary religions, no shaming, no "holier-than-thou" attitudes. Nothing of that kind. We are in this together!

I am not some ivory tower guru. I am a "do-ro," focused on doing (I don't have the time for posing and pontificating), and I am right with you I the trenches (alkaline trenches), moving forward.

My writing style is direct and honest because my biggest goal is to help you transform on a deeper level. And I know that to do that, you need simple to follow and to apply information, backed up with inspiration and motivation to guide you on your journey.

So, inside all of Marta's books- you can feel like at home, and you will not get put down for your nutritional choices, because none of us is perfect. We are in this journey together, and I am very grateful I can be guiding you today!

I had to overcome many physical, mental, and emotional challenges, which turned me into the person that I am today.

This is how real transformation takes place- through overcoming challenges on a day-to-day basis. Nobody is perfect.

I have been living and teaching the Alkaline Diet and lifestyle for over five years now, and it has truly helped me transform not only the way I eat but also the way I live.

I am a self-care advocate and an author of numerous wellness books. I'm a certified holistic nutritionist, aromatherapist, and Reiki practitioner. I have been blessed to be able to study and practice many life-changing natural therapies as well as high performance/ self-development modalities, and I love all of them. Still, the Alkaline Diet lifestyle is undoubtedly one of my favorite tools to share and teach.

The reason I am so passionate about it is that it follows a truly holistic approach and it helps your body restore the balance that it needs to create vibrant health.

It also helps you feel amazing, not only physically but also emotionally. This is a result of increasing your intake of nutrient-rich foods and improving your energy levels. It's also flexible and can be successfully combined with other healthy diets that you may have found beneficial. Yes, it can be combined with keto, intermittent fasting, paleo, vegan...Also, it doesn't require you to go on a crazy, restrictive diet where you are supposed to starve yourself.

That alone is so empowering! People around you will notice your shift and that healthy glow around you. They will want to know your secrets, trust me on that one.

It is my sincere intention that you use this booklet for years to come and discover how much positive change you can create by taking those little inspired, courageous steps every day.

My mission is to inspire you to eat, drink, and live more alkaline so that you can create long-lasting transformation in all areas of your life.

It all starts with health. Some people say, "Health is wealth." I agree, but I would say that health is more than that. Health is life. Value it, put it as your number one priority. Trust me, everything else will fall into place- your family, your career, your finances, and your relationships. With vibrant health comes the courage and confidence to transform other areas of your life and live your true potential the way you were meant to. You will feel so much stronger and courageous!

Let's do this.

I love you; I appreciate you, and I want to thank you once again for taking an interest in this publication and investing your precious time in learning with me.

We're in this together, and I am looking forward to guiding you through this book. I am super excited for you!

Marta "Wellness" Tuchowska

Your friend and coach in Holistic Wellness

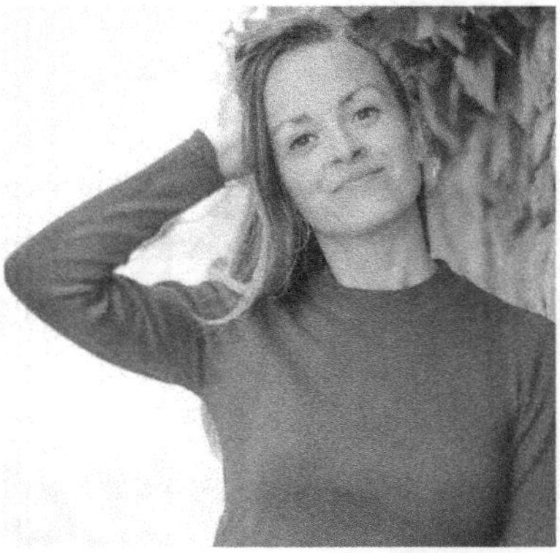

Alkaline Newsletter + Your Bonuses

Before we start our Alkaline Soup adventures, I would like to invite you to join my **Alkaline Wellness email newsletter (it's free).**

When you sign up, you will receive free instant access to 3 **alkaline bonus guides** and **printable food lists** to help you on your journey.

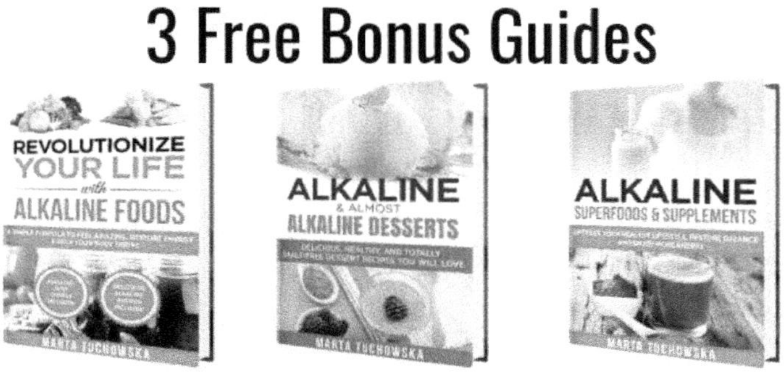

Aside from the 3 bonus guides, you will receive other valuable email updates from me, such as tips and recipes to help you **enjoy your Alkaline Diet lifestyle** and achieve your wellness goals without feeling overwhelmed or deprived.

You will also be the first one to find out about my new book releases, videos, and articles.

You can sign up below via our private, secure website:
www.HolisticWellnessProject.com/alkaline

If you have any problems with your sign-up, please email us at:
info@holisticwellnessproject.com

I honor your privacy and your email box's peace of mind. I will not bombard you with an avalanche of annoying or irrelevant emails.

Only good stuff! I promise. I am a real person, writing real emails to help you and motivate you on your journey. I am not a faceless corporation. And if you don't like me, you can always unsubscribe.

Sign up link to receive your free bonuses instantly:

www.HolisticWellnessProject.com/alkaline

+ the Alkaline Dessert stuff free eBook is the real treat, haha!

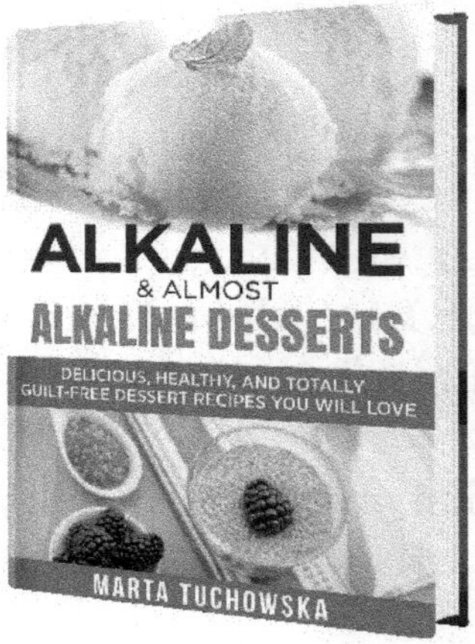

Now, it's time to get down to work and have a look at our alkaline soup food lists and basic shopping lists (flexible and customizable).

Then, we will dive deeper into the alkaline diet and how it works (in case you're new to it or need some refreshment) and finally try the alkaline soup recipes!

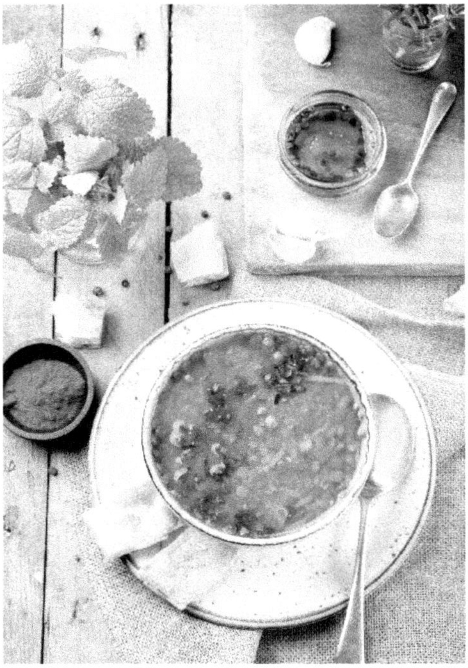

Alkaline Soups- Food Lists

Recommended Alkaline Fruit

As a general rule, the Alkaline Diet encourages you to focus on fruits that are low in sugar. That is why the following fruits are considered super-alkaline:

- Lime
- Lemon
- Avocado (yes, it's a fruit)
- Tomato (yes, it's a fruit)

Yes, acidic-tasting lemons, limes, and grapefruits are actually alkaline-forming fruits (they are alkaline once metabolized).

The simplest explanation for that is that these fruits are very low in sugar and, at the same time, contain alkaline minerals such as Magnesium and Potassium.

While we are not planning on making lemon or lime soups, squeezing in some fresh lemon or lime juice into your soup can make it taste delicious. Especially, if we're making those green, detox soups, or spicy soups...

Tomatoes and avocados are also a must-try for alkaline soups. Avocado will make your soups super creamy and nutritious while adding in some good fats to help you stay full for hours and prevent sugar cravings.

If you need to follow a strict, low-sugar diet because of any medical condition, or a dietary choice (such as low carb or keto), or if your physician has recommended that you reduce all forms of sugar, then, needless to say, it's recommended you focus on super-alkaline fruit (such as fruit low in sugar). And these are excellent alkaline soup ingredients!

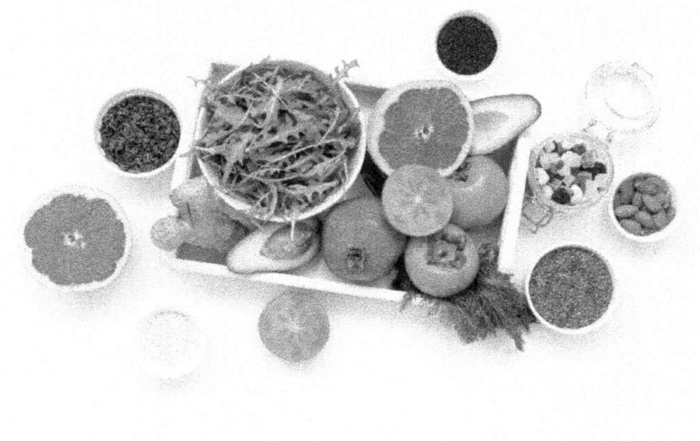

Greens

Greens are very good for you and are super-alkaline.
No worries, they will taste really nice in your soups. The recipes contained in this book have got you covered.

Greens to use in your soups:

- Spinach
- Kale
- Microgreens
- Arugula

+ other fresh leafy greens and greens as well as herbs like:

- Parsley
- Mint
- Chives
- Dill
- Basil
- Cilantro

Alkaline Veggies

All fresh veggies are considered alkaline! So, this one is very easy. One of the goals of the alkaline diet is to encourage you to enrich your diet with more vegetables and greens. The real alkaline superfoods are very easy to find. Nature is all we need to restore vibrant health.

These are my favorite veggies to use in my alkaline soups:

- Red bell pepper
- Green bell pepper
- Yellow bell pepper
- Zucchini (steamed, lightly cooked or raw)
- Broccoli (steamed, lightly cooked or raw)
- Asparagus (steamed, lightly cooked or raw)
- Cauliflower (steamed, lightly cooked or raw)
- Garlic
- Onion
- Cucumber
- Radish
- Artichoke (peeled and cooked)
- Carrot
- Sweet potato (peeled and cooked)

Alkaline Spices & Herbs for Your Soups

The following herbs and spices will make your soups taste original, inspiring, and truly delicious.

- Cinnamon
- Himalayan salt
- Curry powder
- Red chili powder
- Cumin
- Nutmeg
- Italian herbs
- Oregano
- Rosemary
- Lavender
- Mint
- Chamomile
- Fennel
- Cilantro
- Stevia

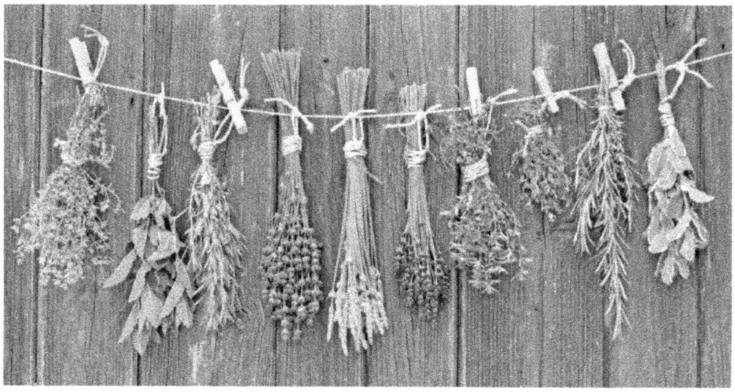

Healthy Alkaline Oils to Add to Your Soups

- Olive oil (organic, cold-pressed) – good for raw or almost raw soups
- Avocado oil – good for raw or almost raw soups
- Coconut oil – good for all kinds of soups, especially oriental, creamy and spicy soups as well as cooked soups and curry style soups.

Alkaline and Almost Alkaline Nuts and Seeds

- Almonds (super-alkaline!)
- Cashews
- Brazil nuts
- Macadamia nuts
- Walnuts
- Pine nuts
- Pistachios
- Hazelnuts

These are also great natural sources of protein and good fats. The most alkaline nuts are almonds (almond milk is also great as we will soon find out). All nuts and seeds are an excellent addition to your soups, but be sure to buy only raw, natural, unsweetened, unsalted nuts and seeds. The reason for this is that processed nuts contain processed sugar and sodium as well as unhealthy, industrial vegetable oils and fats.

Alkaline Friendly Plant-Based Milk and Other Liquids to Use in Soups

As you may already know, dairy is not good for you, and so there is no dairy on the Alkaline Diet. (In this sense, the Alkaline Diet is similar to the Paleo Diet, which also excludes milk and dairy products.)

Most people experience a significantly positive shift in their energy, wellbeing, and vitality just by cutting out (or reducing) dairy from their diet.

For me personally, getting rid of dairy was a big game-changer.

I no longer get any nasty allergies, my digestion has improved, and I no longer feel that annoying burning inflammation in my stomach. Not to mention the fact that I get sick much less, and if I do, I recover very fast. Oh, and my skin is happy too!

I have been living a dairy-free lifestyle for a few years now. Before that, in the first stage of my wellness journey, I studied the macrobiotic diet. I already knew for sure that dairy wasn't my best friend. However, at that time, there was still not that much information on the healthy, plant-based milk options available (aside from soy milk, which, according to the latest research, is not that good for us either).

Luckily, things have now changed, and more and more delicious and nutritious, fully plant-based, healthy milk variations are available even in mainstream supermarkets. Living a healthy lifestyle has never been easier, so if you are only commencing on your journey now, you really should be grateful.

Super-Alkaline Plant-Based Milk

- Almond milk
- Coconut milk

Coconut and almond milk are highly alkalizing and nutrient-packed plant-based milk options.

Some people are allergic to coconut and/or almond milk, or perhaps they don't like them for whatever reason.

If that's the case, there are other options available to help you make delicious plant-based soups.

Other alkaline liquids to use in your soups include:
-clean, filtered, alkaline water
-organic veggie broth or juice

You can also use other plant-based milks such as:
-cashew milk
-gluten-free oat milk
-hazelnut milk
-quinoa milk

These are less alkaline than coconut and almond milk (a staple plant-based milk on the alkaline diet) but are still healthy and nutritious.

My favorites are definitely coconut and almond milk (very alkaline, as well as paleo and keto-friendly). Still, sometimes I also like to use some gluten-free oat milk or other delicious, creamy plant-based milk for more variety.

Just be sure to go for unsweetened, all-natural options with no processed vegetable oils added. (The addition of Himalayan salt is fine.)

The bottom line is- stay away from dairy and experiment with different plant-based milk options too before choosing what works best for you.

The good news is that you can make delicious, creamy, and super tasty soups and creams without using dairy products.

Plant-Based Clean Protein Sources to Use in Your Alkaline Soups:

- Almonds, almond powder, and almond milk
- Quinoa (cooked)
- Pumpkin seeds
- Pistachios
- Flax seeds
- Sesame seeds
- Dark, green veggies (for example, kale and spinach)
- Organic lentils and chickpeas
- Adzuki beans and other beans (organic)
- chickpeas

Extra tip: Be sure to get your free bonus guides and printable food lists by signing up for my alkaline mailing list at:

www.holisticwellnessproject.com/alkaline

Now, it's time for a bit of simple theory.

The hardest part is already behind you because now you understand what alkaline foods look like. So, the next section should be enjoyable and easy to digest. (Alkaline books should be easy to digest, and totally stress-free; otherwise, they are not so alkaline!)

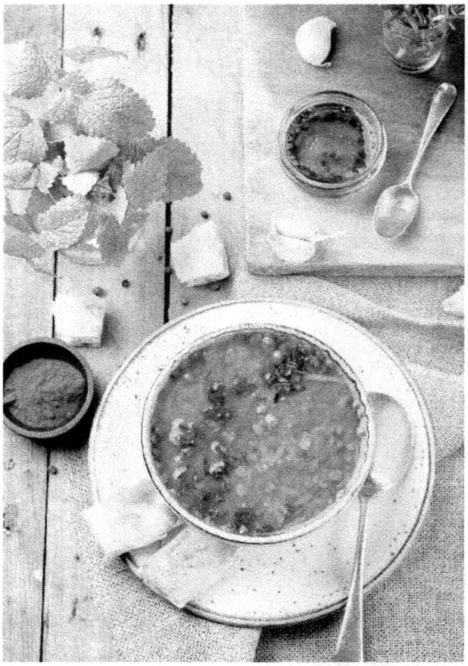

The Alkaline Diet Beginner-Friendly Crash Course

So finally! We get to talk about the pH. Such a hot topic these days!

Luckily, it's much easier than it seems to be...And my goal is to make it as practical and straightforward as possible!

The pH of most of our crucial cellular and other body fluids, like blood, is designed to be at a pH of 7.365, which is slightly alkaline.

Luckily, our miraculous body has an intricate system in place to maintain that healthy, slightly alkaline pH level. It's working for us 24/7, to ensure our pH system stays optimally balanced.

An interesting thing is that our body, as long as it is blessed with the gift of life, will continuously keep working to regulate our pH (whether we eat a healthy diet rich in alkaline foods or not).

The problem? It's up to us to make it easier or harder for our bodies...

We can totally choose what we eat. But...if we focus on unhealthy choices, for example, the Standard Western Diet with its overload of sugars, processed carbohydrates, dairy, soda, too many animal products, and fast food, we make it more and more difficult for our body to stay in balance.

Some people say, "Oh, but what is the point of eating a healthy diet rich in unprocessed alkaline foods if our body regulates our pH for us?"

Yes, our body regulates our pH for us, no matter what we eat. We can't make our pH higher and higher. You see, this is not the goal of the alkaline diet. We just can't make our blood's pH more alkaline or "higher." Our body tries to work hard for us to help maintain our ideal pH. We can't have a pH of 8 or 9. It's not about magically raising or re-modifying our body's pH level.

The focus of the alkaline diet is to give your body the nourishment and the healing tools that it needs to MAINTAIN that optimal pH almost effortlessly.

This is achieved by taking in healthy, balanced nutrition rich in alkaline foods (you already know these are good for you!) such as:

- unprocessed foods
- naturally gluten-free foods (such as veggies)
- yeast-free foods
- dairy-free foods
- sugar-free foods
- wheat-free foods
- foods rich in minerals, vitamins, and chlorophyll
-plant-based foods, greens, and veggies

If we do not support our bodies with healthy, balanced nutrition, we torture them with incredible stress! Yes, when the body has to continually work overtime to detoxify all of the cells and maintain our pH, it finally succumbs to the disease. It still keeps working and balancing...but...it gets weaker and weaker, and we no longer get to enjoy the vibrant health and vitality of our dreams. This is when we become much more prone to disease, and there's a downward spiral of physical and mental ailments.

Let me give a few examples of what can happen if we continuously eat an acid-forming diet (also called SAD - Standard American Diet, or Standard Western Diet) that does not support our body at all. Our body ends up sick and tired of working overtime and may manifest one or more of the following conditions:

- Chronic inflammation
- Immune and hormonal imbalance
- Lack of energy, mental fog- you go for another cup of coffee yet still feel tired....such a horrible feeling..
- Yeast and candida overgrowth
- Digestive damage
- Weakened bones. Our body is forced to pull minerals like magnesium and calcium from our bones to maintain the alkaline balance it needs for constant healing processes.

In summary, eating more alkaline foods, for example, veggies, herbs, and greens helps support our body so that it can work for us at optimal levels. Eating more acidic foods (aka processed food, fast food, sugar, soda, too many animal products, etc.) doesn't help at all. The alkaline diet is not about magically raising or changing our pH, but about helping our body rebalance itself by supporting its natural healing functions with healthy food and drink such as alkaline smoothies and soups.

The commonsense explanation is to imagine you eat a hardcore Western Diet for a month. You eat processed carbs, fast food, drink soda, and bombard your body with unhealthy fats, sugars, and way too many animal products. You don't drink enough water, and you don't move your body. Needless to say, your wellbeing will not improve, and you will begin to feel tired and will very likely have pain and inflammation.

(Fair enough, if you are very young, it may take some time to develop those unhealthy symptoms, but why do that to yourself?)

Then, imagine that you focus on a clean food diet (whether it's fully plant-based, or almost plant-based). You eat lots of vegetables, whole foods, and unprocessed foods. In other words, you eat a diet rich in alkaline foods (and soups!). You also drink lots of clean water, and nutrient-packed smoothies and low sugar juices. Yes, fair enough, every now and then, you have a treat meal or indulge in acidity very occasionally.

However, your overall healthy balance is so strong that your body copes well.

Needless to say, by eating better, by eating a clean food diet and optimizing your health, you feel better and allow your body to heal faster. You treat your body as a temple!

For example, our body also regulates our temperature for us. But...what will happen if you immerse yourself in a bath full of ice cubes for too long? How long will your body keep going and regulate your temperature for you? <u>Everything has a limit.</u>

We can only rely on our "health credit cards" for so long...The first step for most people is to pay off that "health debt." The second step is to make sure your alkaline bank account still has funds in it. The third step is to embrace the Health

Investor mindset. Every food choice we make can be an investment, or an asset, for our long-term wellness, or it can be a distraction/ liability.

The question I ask myself every day is: *Am I getting closer to or farther away from my vision?*

The Alkaline Diet is sisters with the Clean Food Diet, Anti-Inflammatory Diet, Vegetarian Diet, Vegan Diet, Macrobiotic Diet, and the Raw Food Diet. In fact, it offers an incredible blend and the best of them all. All those diets that are more in the plant-based category.

However, what may come as a big surprise to many is that there are also many similarities with Keto and Paleo Diets.

Similarly, to a Paleo Diet (Paleolithic Diet), the Alkaline Diet encourages you to stay away from dairy and wheat as well as processed carbs (such as pasta and "crappy carbs").

Similarly, to the Keto Diet, the Alkaline Diet loves good fats (predominantly in their plant-based version). Also, when it comes to fruit, it encourages you to focus mostly on low-sugar fruit (as we have already covered in the first section of alkaline food lists).

Oh, and again - no nasty, processed carbs. (The Alkaline Diet encourages natural, unprocessed sources of good, healthy carbohydrates that will help you thrive!)

That is why the Alkaline Diet is not just a diet. It's a lifestyle. A nutritionally reasonable, healthily flexible lifestyle that can be combined with other diets you already like and benefit from to make them work even better for you. (Yes, there is Alkaline

Plant-Based, Alkaline Almost Plant-Based, Alkaline Vegetarian, Alkaline Paleo, Alkaline Keto, Alkaline Mediterranean, etc.).

Different strokes for different folks. However, the healthy foundation remains the same: add a ton of alkaline foods into your diet. It's an investment in your health and wellbeing.

What do all the alkaline foods and drinks have in common?

This one is one of my favorite questions. The answer below will help you reverse-engineer different foods to determine whether they are alkaline or not.

As a general rule, all alkaline foods and drinks are naturally
- low in sugar
- gluten-free
- dairy-free
- yeast-free
- high in nutrients (vitamins and minerals)
- plant-based (when going alkaline, you can do a fully plant-based alkaline diet, or reduce your intake of animal products while massively increasing the consumption of plant-based foods – in other words, you can do "almost plant-based," or "mostly plant-based")
- alcohol-free and caffeine-free (no worries, as long as you help your body stay in balance, and you eat and drink healthily, you can enjoy a glass of wine as an occasional treat and some coffee in moderation).
- green -unless they contain caffeine or are high in sugar. For example, green tea is not so alkaline, even though it's green.

(I still use it every now and then, I just enjoy sipping on my green tea!)

Matcha tea isn't, either.

(Again, I still occasionally use it as a non-alkaline part of my diet).

Kiwi fruit isn't very alkaline, but every now and then, I use them in my smoothies or snack on them.

There are many healthy foods and superfoods that are not considered alkaline, and that's OK. The point of the Alkaline Diet (as you will soon find out, or maybe you already know) isn't to eat 100% alkaline all the time. This brings us to the next question...

Isn't it hard to eat alkaline all the time? I like the sound of the health benefits and all that, but I don't think I can eat that way all the time.

The reason I love the Alkaline Diet and have been able to live this lifestyle for over 5 years (and I really enjoy it, get fantastic energy from it and all that) is because of the alkaline 80/20 rule that most alkaline experts recommend. (It works so well!)

The rule is very simple. Your goal should be to make about 80% of your diet alkaline, while the remaining 20% can be other foods. Even 70/30 is an excellent start for most people.

It's as simple as making about three-quarters of your plate full of alkaline foods, for example, veggies. That allows for some flexibility as well as respect for other nutritional choices you may wish to combine with the Alkaline Diet.

You can also start adding alkaline soups to your other meals. Alkaline soups can be a great first or side dish...

Of course, it's all about common sense...The 80/20 rule should not be interpreted as an 80% super-strict, crazy alkaline regime, and 20% eat-whatever-you-want, no limits, fast food, processed junk food.

That would only confuse your body and spoil all the health and wellness efforts you have worked so hard for.
To live this rule with optimum benefit and maximum pleasure, the most reasonable and common-sense thing to do is this:

- Focus about 80% of your diet and lifestyle on delicious alkaline-friendly foods and drinks (fresh salads, more vegetables, yummy soups, satisfying warm alkaline meals, smoothies, greens, juices, ...all the good stuff).

You can get started step-by-step, absolutely pain-free, by combining alkaline foods with "normal food." For example, add an alkaline salad/soup to your regular meal. Alternatively, make a delicious smoothie for breakfast. Start with small goals. Focus first on adding things, focus on abundance.

- Then, for the rest of your diet (about 20%)- add other foods, you feel that your body needs. These may not necessarily be super-alkaline foods, but should still be clean, unprocessed foods as far as possible, including traditional home-cooked meals you like. Within that 20%, a small percentage can be a *now-and-then-indulge-in-some-acidity* treat.

Personally, I love to keep this treat for social occasions and family gatherings. At times like this, I will still drink lots of water, add my alkaline smoothies and alkaline juices and take care of what I like to call "My healthy alkaline foundation."

But...on a special occasion, I will also enjoy a family meal out without worrying all the time about what I eat, or feeling like an alien. I will order my favorite meal with a big bowl of salad, enjoy my time out with family and friends, and the next morning will proceed to make myself a massive alkaline smoothie. Business as usual!

The most important thing is to focus on balance and listen to your body. My goal behind writing this book is to simply inspire you to enrich your diet and lifestyle with alkaline foods and drinks. Oh, and alkaline emotions too...

You see, the Alkaline Diet lifestyle is not only about what you eat, <u>but it's also about how you live...</u>

Stress is very acid-forming, and unfortunately, in this day and age, it's so easy to feel stressed.

Focus on the positive. Take positive action. Love yourself the way you are and never beat yourself up. Respect yourself and your journey. Negative emotions can get us off track. Life can get in the way as things happen. It's normal to experience negative emotions, as well. Nobody is perfect, and in life, we get to experience both positivity as well as negativity.

It's up to us to decide what we focus on. Do not allow anyone to make you feel bad about yourself. Be yourself, think for yourself, choose for yourself.

You can choose to spend more time in nature instead of staying indoors in front of some screen with negative messaging on it. You can choose to read books written by loved-based authors, and you can watch videos that uplift you. You can choose to control your focus.

Ok, enough of my philosophical essays. You are probably thinking, “Hey, just give me those alkaline soup recipes and shut up Marta!”.

But…I always get carried away with this mindset stuff…All practical stuff, not some woo-woo….

The number one takeaway from this section is this: focus on love and kindness as much as you can. That kindness starts with how you treat yourself and who you allow into your mind.

Exploring my mindset and my inner world has been helpful for me and has changed my relationship with food and helped me stay healthy. I genuinely believe in mind-body power and in the healing power of love and positive emotions.

Now back to foods…

What is the difference between the alkaline cleanse and alkaline lifestyle? Do I need to eat this way all the time?

I have noticed that many Alkaline Diet beginners get a bit stuck or confused here, and this prevents them from taking action.

Luckily, it's not that complicated. The Alkaline Diet lifestyle is a simple, balanced, clean food diet combining a healthy lifestyle enriched with a ton of fresh alkaline foods.

It's all about progress, not about being perfect, and it's not about eating 100% alkaline. (Honestly, I don't know anyone who eats 100% alkaline all the time.)

The only exception would be if you are on some specific alkaline healing program (where a strict alkaline eating plan is used), which goes beyond the scope of this book and what I do (this book is not aimed at healing any severe medical conditions).

The basic rule, for an average busy person, wishing to live a healthier lifestyle, is to focus on an abundance of fresh foods, especially veggies, greens, and low sugar fruit. On the Alkaline Diet lifestyle, as you already know, you aim to make about 70-80% of your diet rich in alkaline foods. In contrast, the remaining 20-30% can be other foods.

Still, these should not be processed fast foods. You should always aim for quality, clean eating, so that at least even if it's not alkaline, it's still healthy food.

<u>It's all about balance here.</u>

With such a healthy foundation, it's okay to have some treats here and there, like a coffee (caffeine is not alkaline, I know, I know, what a shame!), a glass of wine or your favorite foods on a family occasion or social get together.

The Alkaline Diet lifestyle can be either entirely plant-based if you want, or it can be combined with other diets, for example, Paleo or Mediterranean ...

It's very flexible, and if you already have another healthy diet that you follow, you can always benefit from enriching your existing diet with more fresh, alkaline foods. This can be done with salads, soups, smoothies, juices, or adding more veggies to your "normal food." That sums up pretty much everything I teach through my books, blogs, and online courses/programs – BALANCE.

However, in some circumstances, you may also benefit from doing an alkaline cleanse...

Ok, so what is an alkaline cleanse? Do I do it?

Yes, 2-3 times a year, I like to go fully alkaline (100% perfect alkaline, haha) for a week or two to restore my energy, getting rid of toxins, and giving my body, mind, and soul a "break."

Alkaline Cleanse – this is when you go fully alkaline for a certain period, usually a week or two, with the intention of deep mind-body detox.

It may also be an excellent solution for those who really need a strong dose of alkalinity to bring their bodies back into balance.

As always, before going on any kind of cleanse, I advise you to consult with your doctor, especially if you are on any medication or experiencing any serious health issues.

Whenever I go on an alkaline cleanse, I nourish myself with 100% alkaline meals, drinks, tonics, and I also drink lots of alkaline juice and smoothies. Yes, I eat 100% alkaline for a week or two (with a short preparation period and after the cleanse period).

During this time, I have no processed foods and no caffeine. This can be a bit difficult if you are hooked on caffeine, but totally worth it because the energy you will get after the cleanse is genuinely amazing!

And a lot of rest while doing this.

Now, while it may sound a bit challenging, for many people, an alkaline cleanse is actually a fantastic experience when appropriately done (enough calories and macros per day, etc.) by following delicious recipes and guidelines.

It's not just about doing some fad cleanse, or a weird one-ingredient detox cleanse. It's about using a variety of different recipes that are 100% alkaline, and that help your body restore all its systems.

Every time I do an alkaline cleanse, I feel stronger, not only physically but also mentally and emotionally, and my nutritional and lifestyle choices get better and better.

After the cleanse, my habits always improve, and I learn a lot about myself and my relationship with food. It feels so good to use food positively as a tool to nourish myself. I feel free to break away from patterns and cravings that do not serve my long-term vision.

The topic of alkaline cleanses goes beyond the scope of this book. That is why I decided to do a little video and an article with extra recommendations, if you would like to explore this topic and go more in-depth:

www.HolisticWellnessProject.com/alkalinecleanse

Now, ...after our super long information + motivation intro, let's dive into the recipes!

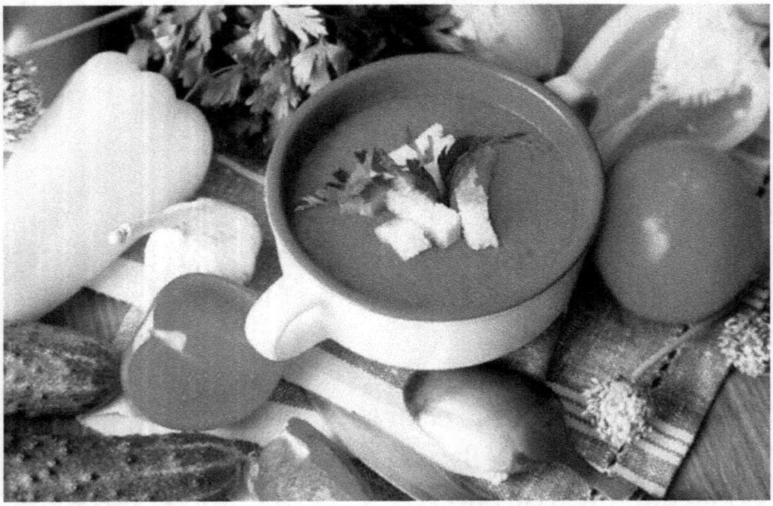

Measurements Used in the Recipes

The cup measurement I use is the American Cup measurement.

I also use it for dry ingredients. If you are new to it, let me help you:

If you don't have American Cup measures, just use a metric or imperial liquid measuring jug and fill your jug with your ingredient to the corresponding level. Here's how to go about it:

1 American Cup= 250ml= 8 fl.oz.

For example:
If a recipe calls for 1 cup of almonds, simply place your almonds into your measuring jug until it reaches the 250 ml/8oz mark.

Quite easy, right?

I know that different countries use different measurements, and I wanted to make things simple for you. I have also noticed that very often, those who are used to American Cup measurements complain about metric measurements and vice versa. However, if you apply what I have just explained, you will find it easy to use both.

Translations (US-UK English)

Eggplant=Aubergine

Zucchini=Courgette

Cilantro=Coriander

Garbanzo Beans=Chickpeas

Navy Beans-=Haricot Beans

Aragula=Rocket

Broth=Stock

About the recipes...

Feel free to customize them. Please don't one star my book, just because one of the recipes called for an ingredient you personally don't enjoy...I didn't put it in there on purpose to upset you, lol! I also have my feelings, haha, and I am a human being! So, let's get together and be all right.

Also, alkaline soup recipes are so simple, that, very often, one of the ingredients can be skipped or swapped.

For example, instead of coconut milk, you can use any healthy plant or nut-based milk of your choice. Or, you can swap kale with spinach or other greens.

Allergic to almonds? Use other nuts instead, or just skip them.

If you have any questions, just email me:
info@holisticwellnessproject.com

Easy Raw (or ALMOST RAW) Alkaline Soup Recipes

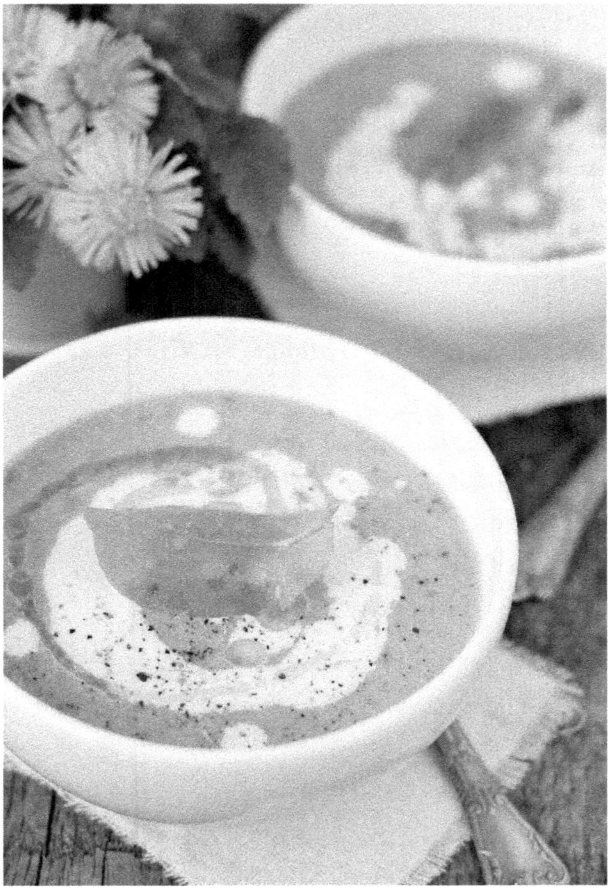

Not a Typical Boring Green Soup

This soup is super rich in nutrients and good fats. But...it's not like typical kale or spinach soup. Instead, it uses cilantro leaves!

This soup is creamy, exciting, aromatic, and fun! It's very quick to make, and it can also be served as a quick side dish.

It can also be enjoyed as a slightly warm, almost raw soup. Just be sure not to overdo the heating process because you want to take advantage of all the fresh and healing nutrients!

Servings: 2-3

Ingredients:

- Half cup fresh cilantro leaves, fresh
- A small handful of fresh parsley leaves
- 1 avocado, peeled and pitted
- Half inch ginger, peeled and pitted
- 2 cups coconut milk
- 4 tablespoons chickpeas
- A big pinch of Himalayan salt
- Pinch of chili and curry powder (optional)

Toppings:

- 1 tablespoon fresh mint leaves, minced
- 2 garlic cloves, minced
- Optional: fried onion rings (if that's your thing)

Instructions:

1. Put everything in your blender and mix until it is completely smooth.
2. Serve with toppings of your choice.
3. You can also serve it with any protein of your choice.
4. Enjoy!

Cilantro is Truly Miraculous!

So, don't be afraid to add it to your smoothies, soups, and salads.

Here are just a few of its benefits:

-improves sleep and reduces anxiety

-adds protection against oxidative stress

-lowers blood sugars

-protects against cardiovascular disease

-makes your skin look much younger!

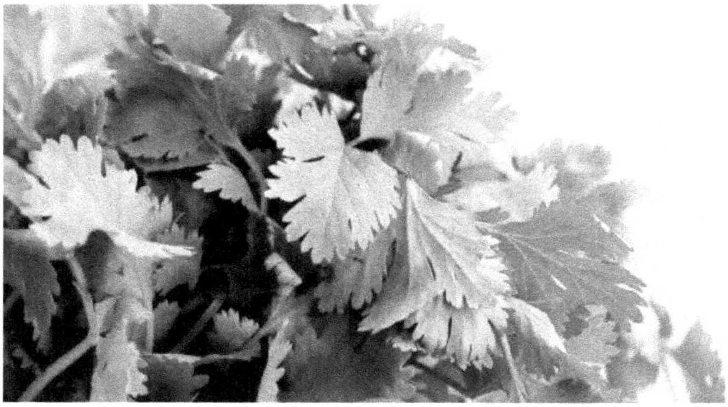

Easy Chilly Beetroot Soup

This soup is creamy, comforting, and very easy to make. It can be served as a 100% raw soup, or lightly cooked.

Servings: 2-3

Ingredients:

- 1 small avocado peeled and pitted
- 1 small beetroot, peeled and chopped
- 2 tablespoons of spring onion, chopped
- 1 small cucumber, peeled
- Half green apple, chopped
- 1 cup water, filtered, preferably alkaline
- Half cup almond or coconut milk

Toppings:

- Fresh dill, chive or herbs like oregano
- Crushed nuts, cashews are one of my favorites!
- Himalayan salt to taste

Instructions:

1. Add all ingredients to a blender.
2. Blend well until smooth.
3. Taste and adjust seasonings if needed. Blend together once again.
4. Serve room temperature or chilled. Add toppings of your choice.

Easy Spicy Coconut Soup

When we think of spicy food, ...what comes to our minds? Probably some yummy curry! And yes, I love yummy, spicy, veggie alkaline curries (you can get a myriad of ideas for these in my book ***Alkaline Diet Spiced Up***).

But...we can also enjoy all those nice, spicy, oriental, and creamy tastes in quick, raw, alkaline soups that take like 5 minutes to prepare!

Servings: 2

Ingredients:

- 2 tablespoons green onion, chopped
- 1 cup thick coconut milk
- 2 tablespoons of curry powder
- 1 minced garlic clove
- 2 small zucchinis, peeled and steamed
- 1 tablespoon grated ginger
- 1 handful cilantro (yes, the famous cilantro makes a comeback)
- 1 green bell pepper, chopped
- 1 small chili flake
- Himalayan salt to taste

Instructions:

1. Blend all the ingredients in a blender or a food processor.
2. Blend 2 minutes to warm the soup.
3. Blend until creamy and smooth.
4. Garnish with cilantro.
5. Serve and enjoy!

Ginger Almond Soup to Fight Sugar Cravings

This recipe is super simple, rich in natural protein and fats, and jam-packed with nutrients to help you fight sugar and crappy carb cravings.

Ginger is alkaline, anti-inflammatory, anti-bacterial, and it will make your soups taste spicy and delicious!

Servings: 2

Ingredients:

- Half cup almonds, soaked in water for at least a few hours
- 1 cup coconut milk
- 2 tablespoons avocado or coconut oil
- Half cup water
- 2-inch ginger, peeled
- Half garlic clove
- 1 big cucumber, peeled
- Pinch of Himalaya salt and black pepper

Instructions:

1. Simply blend all the ingredients in a blender.
2. Serve in a soup bowl (room temperature, or chilled).
3. Enjoy!

A Strong Green Detox Soup for Maximum Energy

This recipe is a real green powerhouse.

Whenever I feel like I need to restore my energy levels, I have this soup for dinner and have an early night.

The next morning, I feel soooo....refreshed! Combining different greens ensures a bigger variety of nutrients...and since this recipe shouldn't take more than 10 minutes to make, putting in some extra effort to get a variety of greens, shouldn't be a problem.

After all, we are investing in our energy. With more energy, we can do more, feel better, and inspire those around us.

Servings: 2

Ingredients:

- 1 small cucumber, peeled
- A handful of baby spinach leaves
- A handful of parsley leaves
- 2 tablespoons of fresh mint leaves
- 2 tablespoons of fresh cilantro leaves (once again, lol!)
- A handful of kale leaves
- A handful of celery leaves
- 1 avocado, peeled and pitted
- 1 garlic clove
- 1-inch ginger, peeled
- 2 cups of coconut milk
- Half cup water, filtered, preferably alkaline
- Pinch of Himalayan salt, black pepper, and chili powder
- 1-2 tablespoons lime and lemon juice to serve

Instructions:

1. Blend all the ingredients in a blender until super smooth.
2. Serve raw, or lightly cooked, if needed.
3. Don't forget to "season" it with some lime and lemon juice (more nutrients and amazing taste!)
4. Enjoy! This one is a true, green alkaline bomb to help you look and feel amazing!

My tip – Green, detox soups like this one, taste great with some thick coconut milk with lime juice. Yummy!

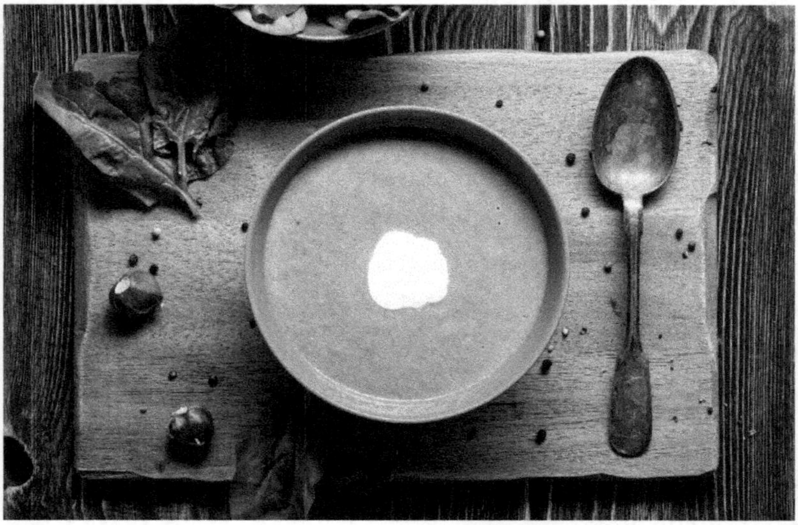

Sweet Potato Almost Raw Soup

This soup combines cooked with raw to help us create balance and enjoy a myriad of alkaline nutrients for optimal energy!

Also, this recipe is very rich in beta-carotene, which makes it an excellent recipe for healthy, young-looking skin! And yea, it's creamy!

Servings: 2

Ingredients:

- 2 big sweet potatoes, peeled and cooked (can be still warm or chilled, it's up to you)
- 2 big tomatoes, chopped
- 4 tablespoons chickpeas (cooked)
- 1 big carrot, peeled and chopped
- 1-inch ginger, peeled
- 1-inch turmeric, peeled (or a pinch of turmeric powder)
- A few onion rings
- 1 garlic clove, peeled
- 1 cup coconut milk
- Half cup water, filtered, preferably alkaline
- Himalayan salt and black pepper to taste
- 1 tablespoon organic olive oil (or avocado oil)
- Optional: cilantro to garnish (it just had to sneak in here!)

Instructions:

1. Put all the ingredients in a blender.
2. Blend well, serve, and enjoy!

Creamy Alkaline Gazpacho for a Healthy Glow

This recipe is inspired by the Spanish Gazpacho recipe. Not only is it rich in beta-carotene and other amazing nutrients to help you have healthy, glowing skin...it's also very creamy and filling!

Servings: 2-3

Ingredients:

- 4 medium tomatoes, skin removed
- 2 big cucumbers, peeled and chopped
- 1 cup coconut or almond milk
- 1 cup water, filtered, preferably alkaline
- A handful of green olives pitted
- 1-inch ginger, peeled and pitted
- 4 tablespoons organic green peas
- Himalayan salt and black pepper to taste
- 2 tablespoons of quality, organic olive oil
- 2 lemon slices, peeled
- Optional: Tabasco sauce to season, if you like it spicy

Instructions:

1. Place all the ingredients through a blender.
2. Blend well, serve, and enjoy!
3. Optional: feel free to serve it with some protein of your choice.

Antioxidant Tahini Energy Soup

Tahini in a soup? Most of us think of tahini as an ingredient typically used for hummus recipes. However, it also tastes great in soups and creams. It's a great way to add powerful antioxidants and healthy fats to your diet.

If you always crave sugar and processed foods, adding more good fats can really make a difference. Tahini is also rich in several vitamins and minerals, such as copper, selenium, and phosphorus, to help you maintain healthy bones, blood vessels, nerves, and immune system while contributing to efficient iron absorption.

Servings: 2

Ingredients:

- 1 large handful of arugula leaves
- Juice of 1 lime
- 1 cup coconut or cashew milk
- Half cup water
- 3 dates, peeled and pitted
- 1 cucumber, peeled and pitted
- 1 big bell pepper, cut into smaller pieces
- 3 tablespoons of raw tahini
- 1 small avocado, peeled and pitted
- Himalayan salt to taste
- Optional: cilantro and parsley to garnish

Instructions:

1. Add all ingredients to a blender. Blend well until smooth.
2. Add more water to or coconut/cashew milk, if needed.
3. Serve and enjoy!

Spicy Celery Gazpacho Soup

Celery is an excellent source of vitamin K, an important nutrient plays a significant role in blood clotting as well as bone and heart health.

It's also a good source of vitamin A (healthy vision and immune system), potassium (one of the most beneficial alkaline minerals we need to stay in balance), and folate one of the B-vitamins. It is needed to make red and white blood cells).

Many people use celery as a juicing ingredient; however, it also tastes fantastic in this spicy gazpacho recipe!

Servings: 2

Ingredients:

- 4 big chopped tomatoes, peeled
- A big handful of celery leaves
- 1 cup coconut milk
- Half cup water, filtered, preferably alkaline
- 1 garlic clove, peeled
- Himalayan salt and chili powder to tastes
- 2 tablespoons chive to garnish
- Optional: you can add in chickpeas or lentils

Instructions:

1. Place all the ingredients in a blender.
2. Blend well until smooth.
3. Serve with some fresh chive and, if needed, add in some lentils or chickpeas.

Alkaline Antioxidant Basil Soup

Remember out little friend, Mr.Cilantro?

Well, this recipe calls for a very similar green ingredient – Mr.Basil! Once again...there are so many greens you can use to create delicious alkaline meals, and basil is one of them.

So, if you are getting bored with spinach and kale, don't worry. There are so many options out there!

Basil is very rich in chlorophyll, and it's also a great source of Magnesium, one of the most precious alkaline minerals. Oh, and it tastes so lovely in soups!

Once again, this soup can be enjoyed raw as well as lightly cooked, the choice is yours!

Servings: 2

Ingredients:

- 1 medium zucchini, steamed, peeled and chopped
- ¼ cup basil
- ¼ cup parsley
- 1 big tomato, peeled
- 1 big green bell pepper, chopped
- 1 cup cashew or coconut milk
- 1 cup of water
- 1 garlic clove, peeled
- Pinch of Himalayan salt and black pepper to taste

Instructions:

1. Place all the ingredients in a blender.
2. Blend until smooth.
3. Serve and enjoy!

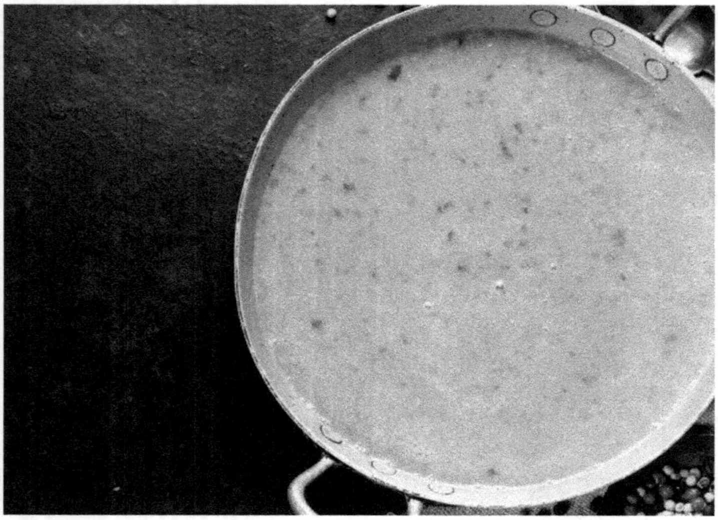

Almost Raw Chili Spicy Tomato Soup

This soup is incredibly simple, and combines the raw with lightly cooked!

Servings: 2

Ingredients:

- 4 big tomatoes
- Half onion, cut into rings
- 1 tablespoon coconut oil
- 1 red bell pepper, chopped
- half teaspoon chili powder
- 1 teaspoon cumin powder
- Pinch of Himalayan salt
- 1 clove garlic, peeled and minced
- Half cup coconut milk, warm
- Half cup chickpeas or lentils, cooked (optional)

Instructions:

1. Put the tomatoes in a bowl filled with hot water.
2. In the meantime, stir-fry the onions in some coconut oil until crispy.
3. Peel the tomatoes and put them in a blender, adding the fried onions.
4. Processed well until smooth and add in the rest of the ingredients (spices, salt, garlic, red bell pepper, and warm coconut milk).
5. Blend again until smooth and serve with some cooked lentils or chickpeas.

Sweet Spicy Soup

This refreshing gazpacho style soup is perfect for hot summer evenings. It blends the sweet with spicy while providing you with a ton of nutrients!

Servings: 2

Ingredients:

- A few pineapple slices
- A handful of cilantro leaves
- 2 small red bell peppers
- half jalapeno, diced and seeded
- 1 tablespoon of lime or lemon juice
- 2 tablespoons of coconut oil
- Half cup of coconut milk
- Half cup of coconut water
- half green onion, chopped
- Himalayan salt to taste
- Optional: crushed almonds or cashews to garnish

Instructions:

1. Simply blend all the ingredients in a blender until smooth.
2. Pour into a soup bowl and sprinkle over some crushed almonds or cashews.
3. Enjoy!

Arugula Healthy Glow Beauty Soup

This simple recipe sneaks in some greens, and it really tastes amazing!

Arugula is great for your skin. This is because it is full of antioxidants and anti-inflammatory compounds.

It is also very rich in alkaline minerals and chlorophyll. Want that healthy glow around you? Add more greens to your diet!

Servings: 2

Ingredients:

- 1 small avocado, peeled and pitted
- 1 small green apple, cut into smaller pieces, seeds removed
- 1 cup cashew or coconut milk (if you can get cashew milk, wow, you're in for a treat! I love cashew milk with this one, however, if you can't get it, coconut milk is fine too)
- 1 cup water, filtered, preferably alkaline
- 1 tablespoon organic olive oil or coconut oil
- A big handful of arugula leaves
- Himalayan salt and black pepper to taste

Toppings:

- Minced onion
- Red pepper flakes
- 1 tablespoon fresh lime juice.

Instructions:

1. Place all the ingredients in a blender and blend until smooth.
2. Add pepper and salt to taste.
3. Place in soup bowls.
4. Sprinkle over some minced onion and red pepper flakes.
5. Spice it up with some fresh lime juice, serve and enjoy!

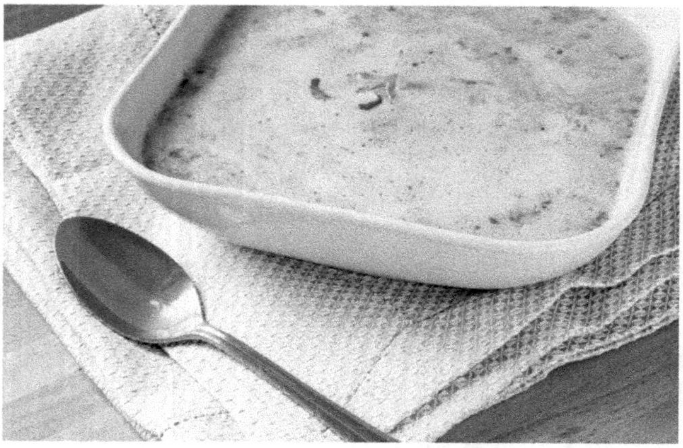

Sweet Dessert Style Creamy Soup

This soup is naturally creamy and sweet and definitely a great choice when you're craving something sweet.

Vanilla and nutmeg add to its natural anti-inflammatory and alkaline benefits.

Servings: 2

Ingredients:

- 1 cup almond milk
- 1 big sweet potato, peeled and cooked
- 1 cup cooked pumpkin
- 1 tablespoon coconut oil
- A splash of vanilla
- A pinch of nutmeg

Instructions:

1. Add all ingredients to a blender.
2. Blend until creamy and smooth.
3. Pour into a soup or dessert bowl.
4. You decide if it's a soup or smoothie.
5. You can serve it chilled or warm, it's up to you!

Sweet potatoes are super nutritious and full of fiber, minerals, and vitamins. They are also rich in antioxidants and help support a healthy vision and beautifully looking skin.

Macadamia Zucchini Detox Soup

Zucchini and macadamia nuts are an excellent blend!

This soup is easy to make, very energizing, and rich in natural protein, good fats, fiber, and plenty of alkaline nutrients!

Oh, and yes, our good old friend, Mr.Cilantro makes a come back once again.

However, feel free to experiment with other greens, such as basil or mint. So yummy, aromatic, and healthy!

Servings: 2

Ingredients:

- 2 zucchinis, steamed and cut into smaller pieces (warm or chilled, it's up to you)
- Half cup macadamia nuts, soaked in water for at least a few hours
- 1 teaspoon organic apple cider vinegar
- 1 lime, juiced
- 1 cup coconut milk
- Half cup water, filtered, preferably alkaline
- Himalayan salt and black pepper to taste
- A handful of fresh cilantro leaves to garnish

Instructions:

1. Place all the ingredients in a blender.
2. Blend well.
3. Pour into a soup bowl, garnish with some fresh cilantro leaves, serve and enjoy.

Ginger Beauty Soup

This is another beta carotene-rich recipe to add to your natural beauty and healthy immune system recipe collection.

It's simple, creamy, and so incredibly aromatic!

Servings: 2

Ingredients:

- 2-inch ginger, peeled and minced
- 2 big garlic cloves, minced
- 1 tablespoon coconut oil
- 2 tablespoons nut butter of choice (personally, I love some fresh, home-made cashew butter)
- 1 cup coconut milk
- Half cup water, filtered, preferably alkaline
- 3 orange wedges
- 3 large chopped carrots

Instructions:

1. Start off by frying the ginger and garlic in coconut oil, using a medium-sized pan.
2. While enjoying the aroma (nothing smells better than stir-fried ginger), proceed to blend the carrots, orange wedges, coconut milk, nut butter, and water.
3. Blend until creamy.
4. Now, add the mixture to the frying ginger and garlic, reduce to low heat, and stir for a few minutes.
5. Serve slightly warm and enjoy!

Simple Warm Recipes

This section will provide you with warm, comforting, filling, chunky style, alkaline-rich recipes.

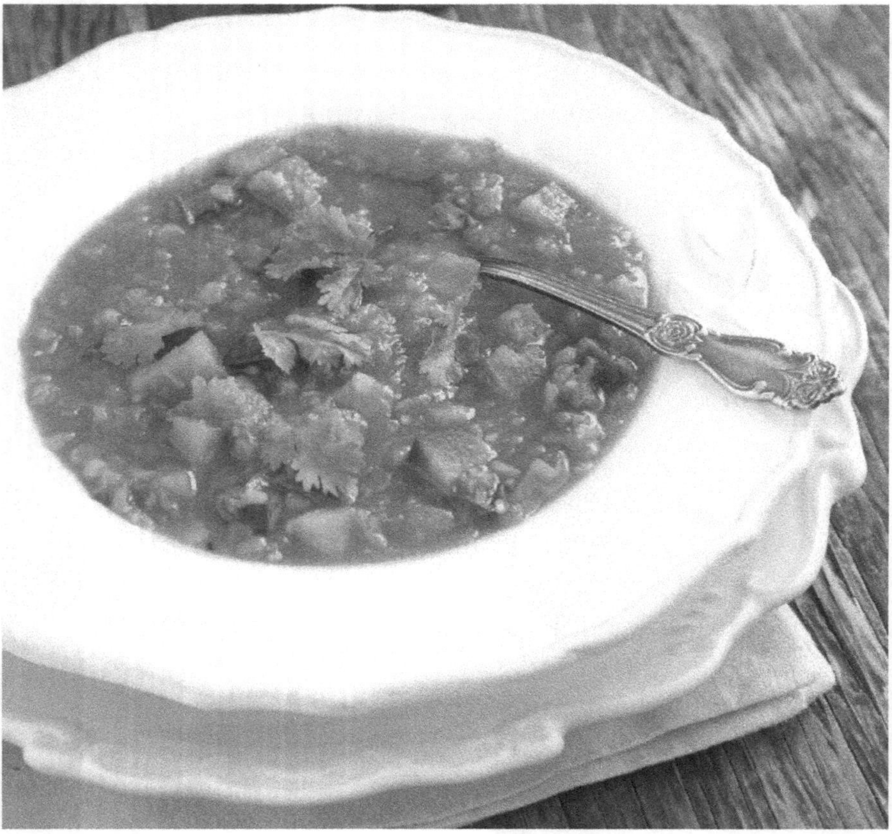

Ginger Comfort Soup

I don't know about you, but I can't live without ginger!

And it's definitely a must-try for warm, comforting soups like this one!

Servings: 2

Ingredients:

- 4 cups organic vegetable broth
- 2-inch piece ginger, peeled and sliced thin
- 1 small red chili flake, minced
- 2 big zucchinis, sliced into smaller pieces
- Half cup chickpeas
- Sliced scallions

Instructions:

1. Put broth, ginger, and red chili in a pot.
2. Bring to boil.
3. Add the zucchini slices and chickpeas.
4. Simmer until the zucchini is tender.
5. Add Bragg liquid aminos.
6. Serve with sliced scallions.
7. Enjoy!

Easy, Filling Rice Noodle Soup

This recipe is a great option to enjoy any time you are craving something Asian. It's simple, spicy, and filling. Oh...and it sneaks in some green veggies too!

Servings: 3

Ingredients:

- 1 big zucchini, sliced
- 1 red bell pepper, sliced
- 1 tablespoon coconut oil
- Half cup white beans, cooked
- 2 garlic cloves, chopped
- A pinch of red chili pepper
- 1 small onion, chopped
- 1 cup organic rice noodles, gluten-free
- 1.5 cup organic vegetable broth.
- 2 tablespoons coconut oil
- Himalayan salt and black pepper to taste
- Fresh lime juice and jalapeno to serve

Instructions:

1. Begin frying the onion in a pan (until golden), using coconut oil.
2. Stir in the garlic and keep stir-frying for a few more minutes.
3. Pour in the veggie broth, add pepper and salt.
4. Add in the pepper, zucchini, and beans.
5. Stir for a few minutes.
6. Now, add in the rice noodles and keep stirring until soft.

7. Take off the heat, stir well, and serve with some fresh lime juice and jalapeno.

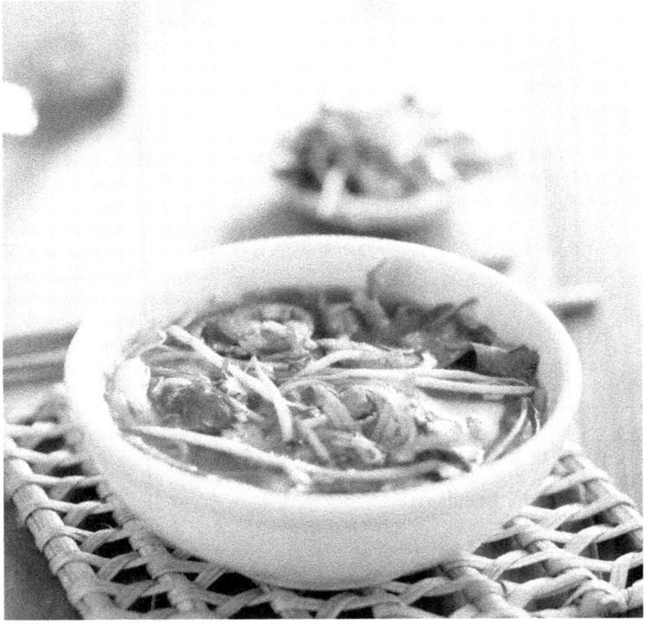

Absolutely Irresistible Coconut Curry

We have already tried creamy curry style raw soup recipes...now it's time for something warm and comforting like this recipe!

Servings: 2

Ingredients:

For the Curry:

- 1 cup organic vegetable broth
- 2 cups coconut milk
- Half cup chickpeas, cooked
- 1 tablespoon coconut oil
- ¼ cup diced tomatoes
- Half cup diced carrots
- Half cup broccoli florets
- 2 tablespoons grated ginger
- 4 cloves minced garlic
- 1 small onion, diced
- Black pepper and Himalaya salt
- Pinch of cayenne and cumin (optional)
- 1 teaspoon curry powder

Quinoa:

- 1 cup quinoa, rinsed
- 1 cup coconut milk

Instructions:

1. Start by prepping the quinoa by rinsing it in a mesh strainer. Toast the quinoa for about three minutes. Pour in a can of coconut milk and a half cup of water. Allow to boil and then reduce to a simmer. Cover pot and let cook 15 minutes. The liquid should be absorbed.
2. While the quinoa is cooking, heat oil and sauté the broccoli, carrot, ginger, garlic, and onion.
3. Season with black pepper and Himalayan salt.
4. Stir frequently until the veggies have softened, around five minutes.
5. Mix in another pinch of salt, coconut milk, veggie stock, cayenne, and curry powder. Let the mixture simmer for about ten to 15 minutes.
6. Stir in the tomatoes and snow peas during the last five minutes.
7. Adjust the taste as needed, adding more pepper or salt.
8. Serve the curry over a helping of the coconut quinoa, as a delicious and filling aromatic soup. Garnish with any herbs that you would like, and squeeze on some fresh lemon juice.

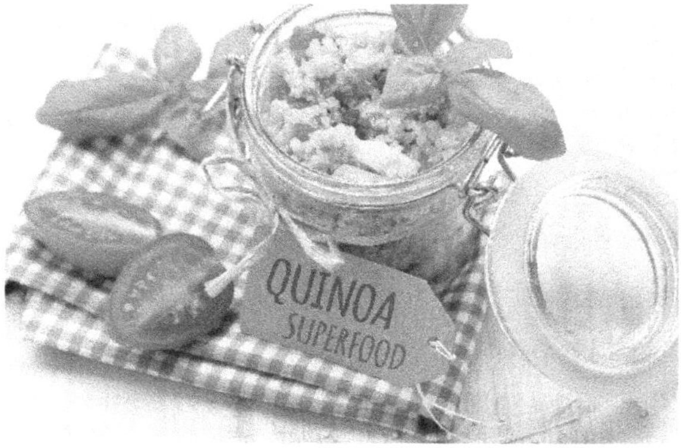

Spicy Moroccan Anti-Inflammatory Mix

This simple soup uses a ton of alkaline herbs and spices such as cilantro, cumin, and allspice.

Not only do they make our soup taste delicious...they also add in some powerful alkaline healing and detoxification.

Whatever meal you are making...heck even if you are making a simple salad or a smoothie...ask yourself if you can also sneak in some herbs and spices.

Yes, cumin also tastes amazing in salads!

If you want to dive deeper into alkaline herbs and spices, I highly recommend you read my book ***Alkaline Herbs***, where I will show you different herbs and recipes for beauty, cooking, wellness, and relaxation.

Now, let's make our Moroccan soup!

Servings: 2-3

Ingredients:

- 2 cups cooked carrots, sliced
- 4 cups organic vegetable broth
- Half cup toasted pumpkin seeds
- Half teaspoon allspice
- Half teaspoon cilantro
- Pinch of red pepper
- Half teaspoon cinnamon
- Himalayan salt to taste
- 3 tablespoons coconut oil

- A big pinch of cayenne pepper
- A big pinch of black pepper
- 1 teaspoon cumin powder
- Half teaspoon ginger powder
- Half teaspoon turmeric powder
- Fresh lemon juice to serve
- Fresh cilantro leaves to serve

Instructions:

1. Add the carrots and broth to a blender.
2. Blend until smooth.
3. Put the mixture in a pot on medium heat.
4. Add in Himalaya salt and spices.
5. Cook for about 10 minutes. Add water until it is at the desired consistency.
6. Serve soup with pumpkin seeds, fresh cilantro leaves, ground pepper, and olive oil.
7. Drizzle over some fresh lemon juice and enjoy!

Italian Veggie Soup

Once again, we are turning to spices and herbs!

They always work like a miracle...even if you are not a veggie person.

This soup is simple, filling, delicious, and smells fantastic! Perfect for cold, winter evenings.

Servings: 3-4

Ingredients:

- 1 cup organic cannellini beans
- 2 cups diced tomatoes
- 2 cups organic vegetable broth
- 1 cup of water, filtered, preferably alkaline
- 1 small broccoli, cut into smaller pieces
- 1 large red onion, chopped
- 1 big zucchini, chopped
- 3 big garlic cloves, minced
- 1 fennel bulb or 4 celery stalks
- Half small butternut squash
- 2 teaspoons of Italian seasoning
- Black pepper and Himalayan salt to taste

Instructions:

1. Start off by blending the beans with tomatoes and vegetable broth using a blender or a food processor.
2. Add pepper and salt to taste, Italian seasoning, garlic, and onion.
3. Bring to a boil and allow it to cook for ten minutes.

4. Add in broccoli, zucchini, squash, and fennel.
5. Simmer vegetables until soft, around 20 minutes, and add more water, if needed.
6. Serve warm and enjoy!

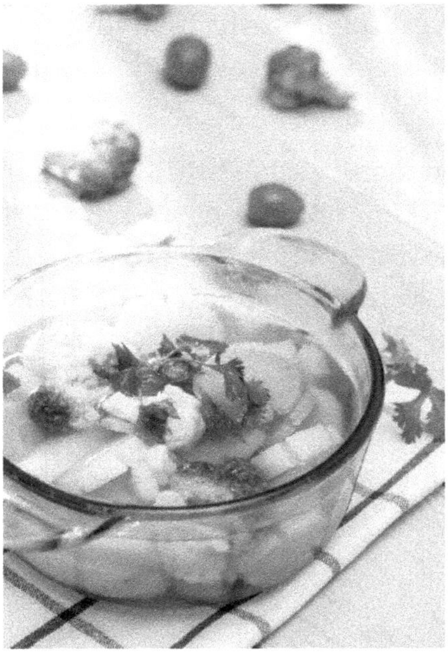

Spicy Creamy Veggie Dream

This recipe is incredibly simple to make. It combines the softness of coconut milk and the comfort of sweet potatoes while adding in a myriad of veggies and even more nutrients via the organic veggie broth.

I am a big fan of vegetable broth! If buying one (I usually do to save time), make sure it's organic, with no added sugar/ no nasty stuff in it.

Sometimes, I even drink veggie broth in between my meals, as if it was water. It's very nourishing and full of minerals. I don't know why, but in winter, I just don't feel like drinking plain water, so I turn to warm herbal infusions, alkaline teas (I got a book on ***Alkaline Teas*** as well if you want to give it a go!) and veggie broth.

And with veggie broth, you can always conjure up delicious soups like this one!

Servings: 3

Ingredients:

- Half cup coconut milk
- 3 sprigs fresh thyme
- 3 medium sweet potatoes, peeled and chopped
- 4 celery stalks, cut into smaller pieces
- 4 garlic cloves, peeled and halved
- 3 cups of organic vegetable broth
- 3 big carrots, peeled and sliced
- 2 red pepper flakes, minced
- 1 large red onion, chopped

- 2 fresh bay leaves
- A pinch of black pepper
- A pinch of Himalayan salt to taste
- 2 tablespoons coconut oil

Instructions:

1. Heat the coconut oil in a pan.
2. Add celery, carrots, and onions.
3. Add some Himalayan salt and red pepper flakes.
4. Cook for about 5 minutes (add more oil if the pan gets too dry)
5. Add vegetable broth and boil.
6. Add potatoes, thyme, bay leaves, and garlic.
7. Simmer until potatoes are tender.
8. Take your soup off the heat.
9. Mix in the coconut milk. Adjust seasoning if needed.
10. Serve and enjoy!

Chickpea Veggie Protein Soup

This comforting soup is full of natural protein and good fats to help you stay full for hours. It also sneaks in some greens and beta carotene-rich tomatoes to help you eat your way to glowing skin and a stronger immune system.

Servings: 4

Ingredients:

- 3 cups organic vegetable broth
- 1 medium red onion, chopped
- Half teaspoon turmeric
- 2 garlic cloves, peeled and minced
- 1 cup water, filtered, preferably alkaline
- 4 carrots, peeled and sliced
- 4 big tomatoes, diced
- 4 celery stalks, sliced thin
- 2 tablespoons coconut oil
- 1 cup chickpeas, drained and rinsed
- 1 bay leaf
- Black pepper and Himalayan salt to taste
- 4 tablespoons thick coconut milk or vegan yogurt (optional)

Instructions:

1. Heat the coconut oil in a pot.
2. Add bay leaf, garlic, celery, carrots, onions, pepper, and salt.
3. Cook for a few minutes.
4. Then, add tomatoes, chickpeas, and turmeric.
5. Stir for a few minutes.
6. Add water, thick coconut milk, and broth. Stir to combine.
7. Keep boiling on low, medium heat.
8. Allow it to simmer for ten minutes. Take off the heat.
9. Taste and add more Himalayan salt if needed.
10. Serve and enjoy!

Sweet Spicy Almond Soup

This soup has got everything you need to stay energized....

Good unprocessed nutrient-rich carbs (nothing to be afraid of!) natural protein and healthy fats, backed up by alkaline, anti-inflammatory spices, and carotene-rich veggies!

Servings: 2

Ingredients:

- A big handful of raw almonds, chopped
- A handful of cilantro
- Half cup almond butter
- 2 cups coconut milk
- 2 tablespoons coconut oil
- 2 garlic cloves, minced
- 2 big tomatoes, diced
- 1 red bell pepper, sliced
- 2 teaspoons cumin
- 1 large onion, minced
- 1 big sweet potato, peeled and chopped
- Half teaspoon cayenne pepper
- 1 tablespoon of fresh ginger, grated
- Black pepper and Himalayan salt to taste

Instructions:

1. Heat some coconut oil in a pan.
2. Add onion, season with pepper and salt.
3. Stir-fry until tender.
4. Add ginger, garlic, cayenne, and cumin. Stir again.
5. Add sweet potatoes and stir to combine.

6. Add the coconut milk, almond butter, and tomatoes.
7. Cover and cook in coconut milk until sweet potatoes can easily be pierced with a fork.
8. Serve the soup with almonds and cilantro.

But I Don't Have the Time to Cook Soup!

This recipe is warm, satisfying, and nutritious. Oh, and it's very quick to make!

Servings: 2

Ingredients:

- 2 thinly sliced scallions
- 1 cup vegetable broth
- Half cup coconut or almond milk (to make the soup creamy!)
- Half cup red beans, rinsed and drained
- 1 teaspoon oregano
- 1 tablespoon fresh lime juice
- 2 garlic cloves, peeled and minced
- Black pepper and Himalayan salt to taste

Instructions:

1. Heat oil in a pan. Add oregano, garlic, and scallions. Sauté until soft.
2. Add beans and broth. Stir. Cook until hot.
3. Add lemon juice. Stir well. Season with pepper and salt.
4. Done! Serve and enjoy!

Extra tip – instead of traditional red beans, you can also use cooked adzuki beans. Adzuki beans are much easier to digest, and they are very often used in Macrobiotic cooking. They taste delicious in this recipe, and in the Macrobiotic diet, they are very often used in the winter season to strengthen the kidneys and get rid of fears and negative emotions.

Coconut Pea Warm Soup

Another super simple recipe that doesn't require hours in the kitchen!

Servings: 2

Ingredients:

- 2 cups thick coconut milk
- 1 cup green peas, rinsed
- Half red onion, minced
- 2 tablespoons coconut oil
- 1 teaspoon cilantro powder
- 1 teaspoon ginger powder
- Black pepper and Himalayan salt to taste
- Lime juice to serve

Instructions:

1. Using a medium-sized pan, stir-fry onion in coconut oil until golden.
2. Add in the cilantro powder, ginger powder, salt, and black pepper.
3. Stir again.
4. Now, add in the peas and coconut milk.
5. Keep stirring on low heat until warm.
6. Take off the heat, pour into soup bowls, serve, and enjoy.
7. Drizzle over some fresh lime juice!

Easy Chickpea Thai Soup

This recipe is super spicy and rich in alkaline nutrients.

It's also very comforting and easy to make – precisely what we want, right?

Servings: 2

Ingredients:

- 1 teaspoon Thai red curry paste
- 1 teaspoon fresh ginger, grated
- 2 cups organic vegetable broth
- 1 cup cooked chickpeas, rinsed
- ¼ cup fresh basil leaves
- 1 cup coconut milk
- 1 cup water, filtered, preferably alkaline
- 2 tablespoons fresh lime juice
- 2 carrots, peeled and sliced
- Chili sauce (optional)
- Himalayan salt and black pepper to taste

Instructions:

1. Mix the curry paste and ginger together in a pot. Pour in the broth and coconut milk.
2. Add a bit of Himalayan salt and black pepper to taste.
3. Stir well until smooth and boil on medium-low heat.
4. Add carrots. Simmer until tender.
5. Now add in the chickpeas and keep stirring.
6. Stir in some fresh lime juice.
7. Turn off the heat.

8. Add in some fresh basil and chili garlic sauce.
9. Serve and enjoy!

Extra tip: after such a spicy meal, you may need some natural refreshment.

Below are my (super alkaline) drink suggestions:

-Fennel tea with some fresh grapefruit juice

-mint tea mixed with coconut water

-rooibos tea mixed with some coconut milk

-fresh lime juice with coconut milk and coconut water

To dive deeper into Alkaline Drinks, I highly recommend you check out my book called...yes...***Alkaline Drinks***!

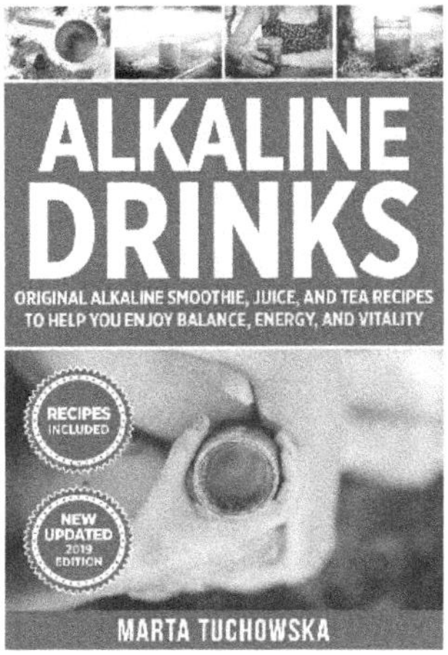

The Kale Queen Soup

Finally, ...the queen of all greens, probably one of the most famous green alkaline food, ever, Miss Kale, made it to the party!

And yes, it tastes great in soups too. Like all greens, it's rich in chlorophyll, and alkaline minerals. The perfect ingredient to help you restore energy, balance, and zest for life!

In this recipe, it also teams up with celery (another super famous green thing) to help us conjure up an amazingly healing and tasty (yes, for alkaline freaks like us!) soup.

Servings: 2

Ingredients:

- 4 stalks celery, chopped
- 1 large onion, chopped
- 1 cup organic beans, rinsed (you can also use red beans, lentils or adzuki beans if you want)
- 1 medium butternut squash, cut into smaller pieces
- Half cup organic, or home-made tomato sauce (or just blend 2-3 tomatoes with some garlic and spices)
- 2 cloves garlic, peeled and minced
- 1 big handful of kale leaves, minced
- 4 cups organic vegetable broth
- 2 tablespoons fresh thyme
- 2 tablespoons coconut oil
- Black pepper and Himalayan salt to taste

Instructions:

1. Heat the coconut oil in a pot.
2. Add the onion, pepper, and salt.
3. Cover and simmer until onion becomes soft.
4. Now, stir in the thyme, garlic, and celery.
5. Let them cook until onion is slightly browned.
6. Finally, add the tomato paste and carry on cooking.
7. Add the veggie broth and squash.
8. Simmer until the squash becomes tender.
9. Add in the kale and beans.
10. Let it cook until kale is tender.
11. Serve and enjoy!

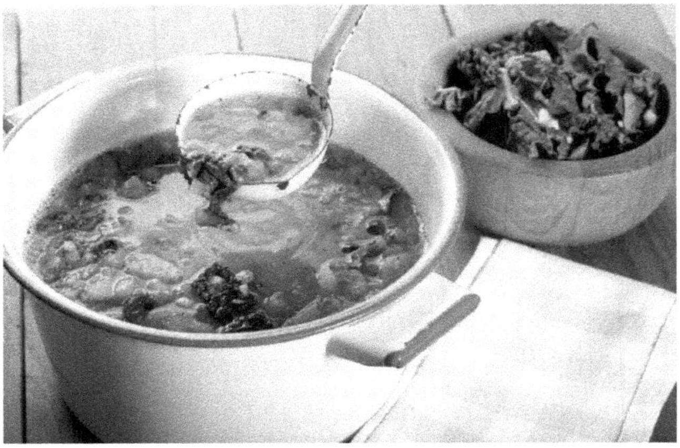

Alkaline Quinoa Dream

Quinoa is an excellent natural, plant-based protein source and will help you stay full for hours. It's also rich in Manganese,

Phosphorus, Copper, Folate, Iron, Magnesium, and Zinc.

Perfect for a balanced, healthy, and alkaline-rich diet (ups...sorry...lifestyle!)

Servings: 2

Ingredients:

- Half cup cooked quinoa
- 2 celery stalks, chopped
- 2 tablespoons Bragg liquid aminos
- 2 cups organic vegetable broth
- 1 red onion, chopped
- 1 teaspoon sweet paprika
- 1 can chickpeas, cooked and rinsed
- 1 big carrot, peeled and chopped
- 1 red bell pepper, chopped
- 2 tablespoons coconut oil
- 3 cloves garlic, minced
- 1 yellow bell pepper, chopped
- A handful of fresh cilantro, chopped
- Black pepper and Himalaya salt to taste

Instructions:

1. Heat the coconut oil using a medium-sized pan.
2. Add the celery, carrots, and onion.
3. Cover. Cook until soft.
4. Add pepper, salt, paprika, and garlic.

5. Add bell peppers.
6. Add the veggie broth and chickpeas. Cook until the vegetables are tender.
7. If needed, add some water.
8. Add in 2 tablespoons of Bragg liquid aminos and quinoa.
9. Serve the soup with chopped cilantro and, if needed, season with more Himalayan salt and black pepper.
10. Enjoy!

Extra Reading:

To learn more about the Queen of this recipe, Miss Quinoa, check out my article:

The Amazing Health Benefits of Quinoa (+ delicious quinoa recipes)

www.holisticwellnessproject.com/quinoa

Spicy Kale & Lentil Soup

This delicious soup is loaded with heart-healthy kale, protein-rich lentils, sweet potatoes, creamy coconut milk, and delicious spices. It's very rich in iron and Vitamin C (great combo!) as well as in alkaline minerals such as Magnesium to help you enjoy more energy, naturally!

Servings: 2-3

Ingredients:

- Half cup lentils, cooked and rinsed
- 1 tablespoon garlic, minced
- 2 small sweet potatoes, peeled and chopped
- 1 small onion, minced
- Half cup kale, tough stems removed and chopped
- 1.5 cup organic vegetable broth
- 1 cup thick coconut milk
- Red pepper flakes to garnish (and make it spicy, if needed)
- 1 tablespoon coconut oil
- Himalayan salt and black pepper to taste

Instructions:

1. Stir-fry the garlic and onion in coconut oil.
2. Add the Himalayan salt and black pepper and continue to cook until slightly crispy.
3. Add the veggie broth and keep cooking on low heat.
4. Add potatoes. Cook until tender.
5. Now, add in the kale, lentils, and coconut milk.
6. Continue cooking until the kale softens up.
7. Serve the soup with red pepper flakes. Enjoy!

Cauliflower Dream Soup

Cauliflower is just perfect for simple, creamy, alkaline soups like this one. It's incredibly hydrating, rich in alkaline minerals, as well as in Vitamin C and Vitamin K.

Servings: 2

Ingredients:

- 2 cloves of garlic, chopped
- 2 cups of coconut milk
- 1 medium cauliflower, chopped
- 1 red onion, chopped
- 2 cups of vegetable broth
- 1 big sweet potato, peeled and chopped
- Black pepper and Himalayan salt to taste

Toppings:

- Curry and other spices of your choice
- Coconut milk, to drizzle
- Olive oil, to drizzle
- Lime juice, to drizzle

Instructions:

1. Combine the coconut milk and veggie broth in a medium-sized pot.
2. Start cooking on medium heat, and add the rest of the ingredients.
3. Feel free to add in any spices you like (for example, curry, chili, cumin, cilantro).
4. Keep cooking until the cauliflower is soft.

5. Taste to see if you need to add more salt or pepper.
6. Pour the soup in a soup bowl, and drizzle over some olive oil and lime juice.
7. Enjoy!

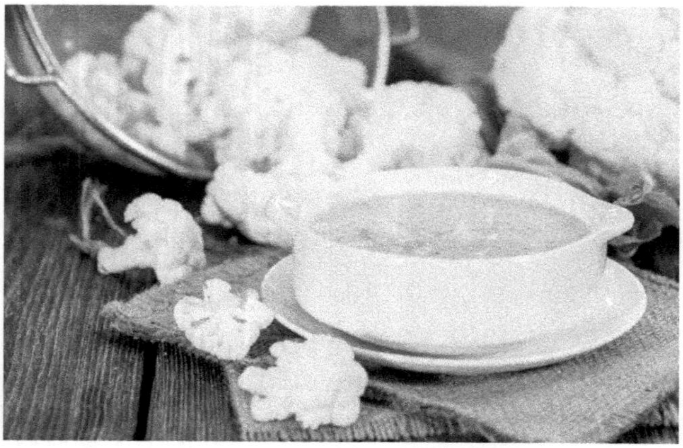

Easy Chunky Veggie Soup

This recipe is simple, comforting, and fun.

It's very rich in alkaline ingredients and spices that do not only make this soup super tasty but also add to its anti-inflammatory benefits.

Servings: 2

Ingredients:

- 1 cup organic green peas, rinsed
- 1 onion, chopped
- 4 carrots, peeled and chopped
- 2 cans of vegetable broth
- 1 cup thick cashew milk (to make it creamy!)
- 2 tablespoons coconut oil
- 3 celery stalks, chopped
- 2 big tomatoes, diced
- 1 teaspoon dried thyme
- 2 garlic cloves, minced
- 2 bay leaves
- A handful of fresh cilantro leaves
- A few mint leaves
- 2 sweet potatoes, peeled and chopped
- Himalayan salt and black pepper to taste

Instructions:

1. Heat the coconut oil in a pan.
2. Add celery, carrots, and onions.
3. Cook a few minutes and add garlic.
4. Add the veggie broth, thyme, bay leaves, cilantro, potatoes, and tomatoes. Season with pepper and salt.
5. Keep boiling and add green beans.
6. Simmer until potatoes are tender.
7. Serve warm and enjoy!

Final Words

Let's finish off this book with my best tips to help you look and feel amazing.

When you combine the following tips with the recipes and empowering mindset from this book, you will be able to dive deep, transform your body and mind, and feel amazing.

Here are a few simple guidelines that will help you transition towards a healthy, alkaline lifestyle. These are compatible with different nutritional lifestyles (Gluten-Free, Vegetarian, Vegan, Paleo, you name it!), and it's totally up to you what you choose to focus on.

Tip#1....

Eliminate processed foods from your diet and say "no" to colas and sodas

There are so many additives and preservatives in these foods. They have been known to create hormone imbalances, make you tired, and add to acidity in your body. It's just not natural for humans to consume those conveniently processed foods.

The label may even say "low in calories or low in fat," but it will not help you in your long-term weight loss or health efforts. To start losing weight naturally, your body needs foods that are jam-packed with nutrients. Real foods. Living foods.

Add more raw foods to your diet.

Focus on adding lots of vegetables and leafy greens as well as fruits that are naturally low in sugar (for example, limes, lemons, grapefruits, avocados, tomatoes, and pomegranates are alkaline-forming fruits).

Reduce/eliminate animal products

These are very acid-forming. The good news is that there are many plant-based options out there and tons of ways to create delicious alkaline-friendly plant-based meals you will love!

Whether you want to eat fully plant-based, or almost plant-based, or you simply want to eat more vegetables, it's your decision, so I am not here to preach the exact way you "should" be eating.

But...even by making most of your diet alkaline plant-based, you will begin to feel lighter and more energized. Also, plant-based recipes are creative and inexpensive.

Drink plenty of clean, filtered water

Preferably drink alkaline water or alkaline fruit-infused water (lemons, grapefruits, limes, and pomegranates are great for that).

Add more vegetable juices into your diet.

These are a great way to give your body more nutrients and alkalinity that will result in more energy, less inflammation, and, if desired, natural weight loss.

Vegetable juices are the best shots of health! I have also written a book called ***Alkaline Juicing*** if you want to give it a try and want to learn how to juice the right way, to enjoy more energy and health.

Reduce/eliminate processed grains, "crappy carbs," as well as yeast (very acid-forming).

Personally, I recommend quinoa instead (it's naturally gluten-free), some sweet potatoes, or some fresh seasonal fruit.

You can also use gluten-free wraps or make your own bread.

Reduce/eliminate caffeine

Trust me - it will only make you feel sick and tired in the long run and can even lead to adrenal exhaustion or chronic fatigue.

It may seem a bit drastic at first, and yes, I know what you're thinking- there are so many articles out there praising the benefits of caffeine and coffee.

Yes, I am sure there are, as many people build their business around coffee. That is why there must be something out there that promotes it. At the same time, I agree that everything is good for you in moderation.

As long as you have a healthy foundation, you can have coffee as a treat.

There is no reason to be too strict on yourself, just don't rely on caffeine as your primary source of energy. Green tea may be helpful also as a transition, but green tea is not caffeine-free either, so don't overdo it.

On the other end of the spectrum - green tea is rich in antioxidants and a great part of a balanced diet, so it's not that you have to get paranoid about all kinds of caffeine. Moderation is key.

Try to observe your body. Personally, I have noticed that quitting my coffee habits (I used to have 2-3 coffees a day) and replacing coffee with natural herbal teas and infusions has really made my energy levels skyrocket.

Now I sleep better, and I get up feeling nice and fresh. I don't need caffeine to keep me awake. I no longer suffer from tension headaches, and I feel calmer.

Yes, I do have a cup of coffee as a treat sometimes, usually when I meet with a friend for a chat, but I no longer depend on it. I choose it; it doesn't choose me.

Think about this and how you can apply this simple tip to your life to achieve total wellbeing. Coffee and caffeine, in general, are very acid-forming.

I recently started using an Ayurvedic herb called Ashwagandha. It is known as an adaptogenic herb, and it can help you restore your energy levels naturally (be sure to consult it with your doctor first, just like in the case of any herb, supplement, or natural therapy).

I have also written a book called ***Alkaline Teas***. It's all about healing, herbal, alkaline friendly infusions that will help you get your energy naturally so that you don't need to depend on caffeine. In this book, I go deeper into no caffeine drinks. Even skipping your normal cup of coffee here and there and going for a nice herbal infusion now and again can really add to your natural energy levels.

Replace cow's milk with almond milk, coconut milk or any other plant-based friendly milk

As you already know, cow's milk is extremely acid-forming. Personally, I don't think it makes sense for humans to drink milk that is naturally designed for fattening baby calves, not humans. Quitting dairy is one of the best things I have done for myself.

I have noticed that even very little milk would cause digestive problems, and it was really easy to fix-I quit drinking milk.

The best thing about the alkaline plant-based diet is that you can still have ice cream and other treats- you just make them with no milk/animal products.

It's so much healthier and tastier, totally guilt-free. With this approach, there is no need to go hungry or be deprived.

Go to www.holisticwellnessproject.com/alkaline

To grab a free copy of my exclusive e-book "Alkaline Desserts" for unlimited healthy treat and dessert ideas.

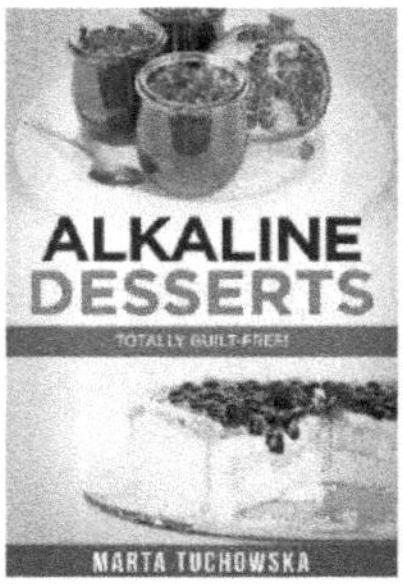

Don't fear good fats- quality coconut oil, olive oil, avocado oil, etc.

These alkaline oils are good for you and should replace processed margarines, and artery-clogging trans-fats. This is not to say that you can "drink" them freely. Balance is the key.

Use stevia instead of processed sugar and Himalayan salt instead of regular salt.

Stevia is sweet but sugar-free, and Himalayan salt contains calcium, iron, potassium, and magnesium, plus it also contains lower amounts of sodium than regular salt.

Add more spices and herbs to your diet- not only do they make your dishes taste amazing, but they also have anti-inflammatory properties and help you detoxify (cilantro, turmeric, and cinnamon are miraculous).

As you can see, the Alkaline Diet is a pretty common-sense clean diet. Nothing is exaggerated. Nothing is too strict. Nothing is too faddish. Eat more living foods and avoid processed foods. Try to eat more plant-based foods (even if you're not fully vegan).

Add regular relaxation techniques to the Alkaline Diet (including yoga, meditation), time spent in nature, adequate sleep, and physical activity (we need to sweat out those toxins), and you have a prescription for health.

It's strange to me that there are so many people putting the Alkaline Diet down. However, the general guidelines I have mentioned above are common sense for a healthy lifestyle, and I am sure your doctor would agree with it (more natural foods, less processed junk, eat more veggies, drink more water, add more relaxation, reduce/manage stress).

This is the gist of the Alkaline Diet lifestyle. This is what will make you feel fresh and rejuvenated and help you achieve your ideal weight. The problem is that some people are not willing to take those small common-sense steps and are looking for a "secret formula"- something that will magically help them with no effort at all. I am not judging- I have been guilty of it as well. We all have! The truth is that whatever changes you want to make in your life (this rule applies not only to health) can be hard. Leaving one's comfort zone is difficult, but with time and practice, it becomes smooth and automatic.

Holistic success is about applying what we already know and using the information to better our lives. This is what I call "the secret formula." Information in action. I always say that I am very open-minded when it comes to different diets. I never claim that what I do is the only path to wellness and health. I prefer to provide you with information and inspiration so that you can create your own way and choose what works for you. Everyone is different. You need to learn to listen to your body and be kind to yourself. Everyone is different, which is why your alkaline lifestyle will be different from mine. However, many elements remain similar, and it is my hope that this book has given you the tools, recipes, and inspiration you need to be successful in your health and wellness quest.

Feel free to come back to this book whenever you need more motivation. It's all about making consistent progress and about those small daily decisions. They will help you create what I like to call *empowering mini alkaline habits*. These, when compounded, will help you to transform in a way you never even thought was possible. It will be a fantastic experience.

Finally, I need to ask you for a small favor. It will only take a few minutes of your precious time and will be very helpful for me at this stage. All I am asking you for is your honest review on Amazon.

Your review, even a short one, can inspire someone else to start living a healthy lifestyle and enjoy the benefits of alkaline soups.

Thank you, thank you, thank you. I am really looking forward to reading your review. Wishing you all the best on your holistic wellness journey,

Marta

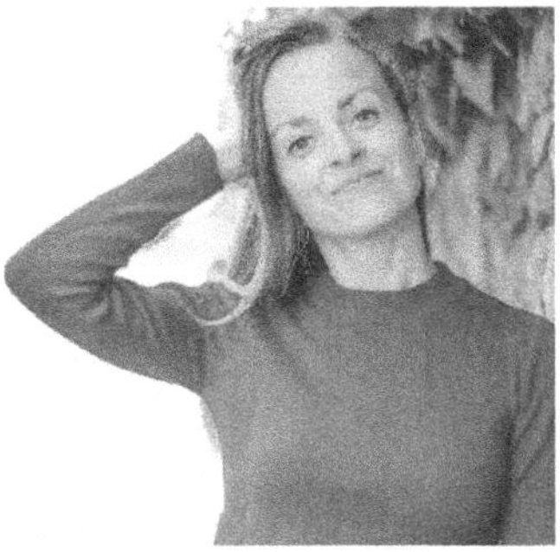

Let's Connect

1. Join my Alkaline Wellness Newsletter and get free instant access to my best tips and recipes, inspiring emails to help you stay on track, as well as 3 bonus guides, simple alkaline food lists and much, much more:

   www.HolisticWellnessProject.com/alkaline

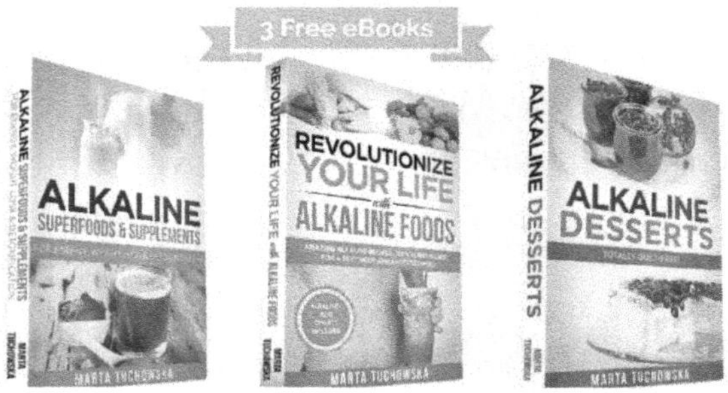

2. Follow my blog posts for more inspiration, motivation and recipes:

   www.HolisticWellnessProject.com/blog

3. My email (in case you want to say *Hi*): info@holisticwellnessproject.com

As I am writing this, I am on a big social media detox. I find it very alkaline! I think I can add more value to you by creating more blog posts or books like this one, and so as of now, I am not active on Instagram/ social media platforms. So, if you need anything- just email me.

My books, courses, and recommendations:

Books: www.HolisticWellnessProject.com/books

Courses: www.AlkalineDietLifestyle.com

My recommendations (diet, tools, supplements, programs, natural remedies):
www.HolisticWellnessProject.com/resources

4. Follow my work on Amazon to get notified about my new book releases and other deals:

   www.amazon.com/author/mtuchowska

Lightning Source UK Ltd.
Milton Keynes UK
UKHW021859280620
365591UK00014BA/719

9 781913 575892